PSYCHIATRY – THEORY, APPLICATIONS AND TREATMENTS

DEPRESSION AND ANXIETY

PREVALENCE, RISK FACTORS AND TREATMENT

PSYCHIATRY – THEORY, APPLICATIONS AND TREATMENTS

Additional books and e-books in this series can be found on Nova's website under the Series tab.

PSYCHIATRY – THEORY, APPLICATIONS AND TREATMENTS

DEPRESSION AND ANXIETY

PREVALENCE, RISK FACTORS AND TREATMENT

SHELLEY L. BECKER
EDITOR

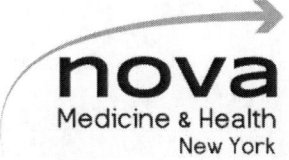

Copyright © 2020 by Nova Science Publishers, Inc.

All rights reserved. No part of this book may be reproduced, stored in a retrieval system or transmitted in any form or by any means: electronic, electrostatic, magnetic, tape, mechanical photocopying, recording or otherwise without the written permission of the Publisher.

We have partnered with Copyright Clearance Center to make it easy for you to obtain permissions to reuse content from this publication. Simply navigate to this publication's page on Nova's website and locate the "Get Permission" button below the title description. This button is linked directly to the title's permission page on copyright.com. Alternatively, you can visit copyright.com and search by title, ISBN, or ISSN.

For further questions about using the service on copyright.com, please contact:
Copyright Clearance Center
Phone: +1-(978) 750-8400   Fax: +1-(978) 750-4470   E-mail: info@copyright.com.

NOTICE TO THE READER

The Publisher has taken reasonable care in the preparation of this book, but makes no expressed or implied warranty of any kind and assumes no responsibility for any errors or omissions. No liability is assumed for incidental or consequential damages in connection with or arising out of information contained in this book. The Publisher shall not be liable for any special, consequential, or exemplary damages resulting, in whole or in part, from the readers' use of, or reliance upon, this material. Any parts of this book based on government reports are so indicated and copyright is claimed for those parts to the extent applicable to compilations of such works.

Independent verification should be sought for any data, advice or recommendations contained in this book. In addition, no responsibility is assumed by the Publisher for any injury and/or damage to persons or property arising from any methods, products, instructions, ideas or otherwise contained in this publication.

This publication is designed to provide accurate and authoritative information with regard to the subject matter covered herein. It is sold with the clear understanding that the Publisher is not engaged in rendering legal or any other professional services. If legal or any other expert assistance is required, the services of a competent person should be sought. FROM A DECLARATION OF PARTICIPANTS JOINTLY ADOPTED BY A COMMITTEE OF THE AMERICAN BAR ASSOCIATION AND A COMMITTEE OF PUBLISHERS.

Additional color graphics may be available in the e-book version of this book.

Library of Congress Cataloging-in-Publication Data

Names: Becker, Shelley L., editor.
Title: Depression and Anxiety: Prevalence, Risk Factors and Treatment
Description: New York: Nova Science Publishers, [2019] | Series: Psychiatry – Theory, Applications and Treatments | Includes bibliographical references and index.
Identifiers: LCCN 2019957633 (print) | ISBN 9781536172294 (paperback) |
  ISBN 9781536172300 (adobe pdf)

Published by Nova Science Publishers, Inc. † New York

CONTENTS

Preface		vii
Chapter 1	On a Path to Integration of the Theory and Practice of Depression: Evolution, Stress, and Predictive Processing *Valery Krupnik*	1
Chapter 2	Sexual Dysfunction and Depression in Females *Swaleha Mujawar, Suprakash Chaudhury and Daniel Saldanha*	57
Chapter 3	A Comparative Study of the Use of Benzodiazepines among Patients with Major Depression and Anxiety Disorders *María Yoldi-Negrete, Rebeca Robles-García, Nicolás Martínez-López, Sara Martínez-Camarillo, Mariana Jiménez-Tirado, Carlos-Alfonso Tovilla-Zárate, Eduardo Madrigal and Ana Fresán*	83

Chapter 4	Immunology of Anxiety Disorders *Suprakash Chaudhury, Satyam Kishore,* *Ajay K. Bakhla and Swalwha Mujawar*	**103**
Chapter 5	Psychophysiological Measures of Anxiety *Suprakash Chaudhury, Swaleha Mujawar* *and Daniel Saldanha*	**123**
Index		**135**
Related Nova Publications		**141**

PREFACE

Depression has always been at the center stage of psychiatry, with many resources allocated to its study and treatment. *Depression and Anxiety: Prevalence, Risk Factors and Treatment* first reviews the emerging Integrative Evolutionary-Stress Response-Predictive Processing Framework Theory, which may offer useful insights for clinical practice.

Sexual problems and dissatisfaction with sex are commonly associated with depression. More awareness and a better understanding of this condition can lead to effective treatment and enhancement of quality of life.

Following this, the authors compare benzodiazepine use in patients with major depression and anxiety disorders to determine which demographic features are related to benzodiazepine use and constitute risk factors for benzodiazepine dependence.

Literature suggests correlations between the abnormalities in the hypothalamic–pituitary–adrenal axis and anxiety disorders, especially in terms of cortisol levels. As such, this compilation systematically assesses the available research data in the last 10 years, shedding light on the association between psychoneuroimmunology and anxiety.

The closing article uses pooled data from 1983-2008 to assess the psychophysiological measures of anxiety. Various databases were searched for articles in English using search words related to psychophysiological measures of anxiety, markers for anxiety, physiological changes anxiety, and monitors of emotional change. The implications of the findings will contribute to further research on improved management for anxiety disorders.

Chapter 1 - Depression has always been at center stage of psychiatry with many resources allocated and a significant progress made in its study and treatment. Still, it remains a wide-spread condition afflicting about 5-10% of the world population and is the leading cause of disability. Depression is a heterogeneous condition with multiple manifestations, symptoms, comorbidities, and degrees of severity compounding the challenge to its treatment. In this chapter, the author suggests that progress in understanding the nature of depression and development of its general theory may assist further advancements in its therapy. Evolutionary theory of depression has developed over several decades and is currently entrenched in the clinical thinking. More recently, a novel paradigm known as predictive coding (or predictive processing framework, PPF) has been proposed as a theoretical frame for understanding psychopathology including depression. PPF has been used as a conceptual bridge linking evolutionary and stress theories to explain mood/affective psychopathology. This emerging *Integrative Evolutionary-Stress response-PPF* (iESP) theory may offer useful insights for clinical practice. The author reviews the rationale and recent developments in this integrative endeavor and discuss how the integrated perspective on depression can guide its treatment. To illustrate this with a clinical example, the author presents a novel evolutionary-based integrative therapy for depression.

Chapter 2 - A detailed search of the medical literature was conducted and articles from 1997-2009 were studied. Search methods included MEDLINE and PubMed databases for articles in English using search words of sexual dysfunction females/women, depression and depression and female sexual dysfunction. A total of 204 articles were screened for inclusion. Sexual problems and dissatisfaction with sex were commonly associated with depression. The prevalence of sexual problems in patients with depression is approximately twice that of the controls. Some of the antidepressants prescribed for depression may lead to impairment in the sexual functioning in all the phases of the sexual cycle. Antidepressant induced sexual problems become a significant concern in the situation of management effectiveness, as antidepressants are useful only as long as the patient takes them regularly. Unbearable adverse effects can be one reason that patients do not take medicines or stop them abruptly. However, most of the studies of drug induced sexual dysfunctions have combined data together for both males and females, barring a few. The implications of the findings will create more awareness and a better understanding of this condition and lead to effective treatment and enhancement of quality of life.

Chapter 3 - *Introduction*. Benzodiazepines (BZDs) are some of the most frequently prescribed psychotropic medications in the world. Under proper prescription, BZDs have sedative and antianxiety properties useful for specific purposes in the treatment of several mental conditions, such as anxiety disorders and depression. For depression, BZDs are not routinely indicated due to their lack of antidepressant effect, but their short-term use may be helpful when depression displays severe anxiety symptoms. In general, as stated in several clinical guidelines and expert consensus, it is recommended the short-term use of BZDs and a continuous clinical monitoring of their use, as the long-term use may be associated to several complications, including dependence and worsening of the underlying condition.

The present study aims to contribute to the body of knowledge about BZDs use in middle-income countries, such as Mexico, where an important number of patients with anxiety disorders and depression are treated for prolonged periods with BZDs. Therefore, the objective was to compare BZD use between patients with major depression and anxiety disorders (generalized anxiety disorder and panic disorder) to determine which demographic features are related to BZD use and constitute risk factors for BZD dependence.

The authors hypothesize that both groups will report a prolonged time of BZDs use, and more patients with anxiety disorders will exhibit BZD dependence; while being a woman, having an older age, being single, with a more prolonged use of BZDs and having an anxiety disorder will be risk factors for BZD dependence.

Method. A total of 158 patients were recruited from the outpatient service at a highly specialized psychiatric facility in Mexico City. Patients were included if they were over 18 years of age and met DSM-IV criteria for major depression, generalized anxiety disorder or panic disorder without any other significant comorbidity and were current BZDs users.

Diagnosis of major depression and anxiety disorders (generalized anxiety disorder and panic disorder) were determined with the Structured Clinical Interview for DSM-IV Axis I Disorders (SCID-I). Also, to determine BZD dependence, an adapted version of the substance dependence section of the SCID-I designed to assess BZD use exclusively was used. Demographic features and characteristics of BZD use of each patients were obtained by a face-to-face interview with the patient. To assess the subjective experience with BZDs in the last month, the Benzodiazepine Dependence Questionnaire in its Mexican version (BDEPQ-MX) was used.

For the comparison between groups chi square tests and independent samples t Tests were used while two multivariate logistic regression models with the backward conditional method were used to determine risk factors associated to BZD dependence in patients with depression and anxiety disorders.

Results. From the patients included, 55.7% (n = 88) had an anxiety disorder and the remaining 44.3% (n = 70) were diagnosed with major depression. Women accounted for most patients with depression (82.9% vs. 69.3%) while patients with anxiety disorders were younger (50.4 vs. 56.1 years). Patients with anxiety disorders had an earlier onset of BZD use (39.7 vs. 46.6 years). Insomnia, as the main reason for BZD use was reported in 47.1% (n = 33) of patients with depression and only in 20.5% (n = 18) of patients with anxiety disorders. BZD dependence was more frequently observed in patients with anxiety disorders (58.0% vs. 41.4%). No differences between groups were observed in terms of the subjective experience with BZD assessed with the BDEPQ-MX. Time of consumption was over 7 years for both groups.

The results of the logistic regression models showed that time of consumption was a risk factor for BZD dependence in both groups, while protective factors for BZD dependence included being a male in patients with anxiety disorders, and being younger for patients with depression

Discussion. In present study, several differences between patients with major depression and anxiety disorders related to BZD use were found. Long-term use of BZDs was observed in both groups and was the main predictor for BZD dependence. Although the presence of anxious symptoms was the most frequent reason for BZD prescription, an important percentage of patients with depression use these medications for insomnia, which may expose the patients to several risks associated to BZD use.

Safety and efficacy of the long-term use of BZD has been subject of controversy. Restriction in prescription may also be ineffective as BZDs may be prescribed repeatedly, resulting in long-term use.

Further studies assessing safety and effectiveness, as well as efforts to encourage and train clinicians and patients to use other alternative medications and non-pharmacological interventions for symptoms where BZDs are prescribed, such as anxiety and insomnia, are necessary to develop complementary treatments without the clinical risks associated to BZDs use.

Although the effectivity of BZDs has been proved, clinicians and patients should establish clear and specific goals for their use since the initial treatment plan for depression and anxiety disorders.

Chapter 4 - There has been increasing focus placed on immune mediated theories in understanding the underlying mechanisms of disorders like anxiety, posttraumatic stress, and obsessive compulsive disorders as the prevalence of these disorders continues to rise all over the world. Literature suggests correlations between the abnormalities in the hypothalamic–pituitary–adrenal (HPA) axis and these disorders, especially in terms of cortisol levels. This chapter systematically assesses the available research data in the last 10 years which sheds light on association between psychoneuroimmunology and anxiety. Finding out the underlying processes leading to these illnesses is crucial for specific and effective treatment strategies, giving rise to considerable improvement in overall functioning, and also considerable decreases in burden on the economy and society.

Chapter 5 - This chapter uses pooled data from 1983-2008 to assess the psychophysiological measures of anxiety. Various databases were searched for articles in English using search words of psychophysiological measures of anxiety, markers for anxiety, physiological changes anxiety, and monitors of emotional change. A total of 76 articles were screened and the bibliographies of all relevant articles were searched for further publications. It was found that anxiety leads to sympathetic over-activity which can be measured by heart-rate, blood-pressure electroencephalogram etc. Loudness of the auditory evoked potential measures activity in the primary auditory cortex in response to different tone intensities and is inversely proportional to serotonergic activity. Patients with anxiety disorders have reduced heart rate variability. The serotonin transporter promoter polymorphism is another measure. Individuals carrying one or two copies of the 's' form had reduction in 5-HTT availability and were associated with increased anxiety. The implications of the findings will contribute to further research and development of better management for anxiety disorders.

In: Depression and Anxiety
Editor: Shelley L. Becker

ISBN: 978-1-53617-229-4
© 2020 Nova Science Publishers, Inc.

Chapter 1

ON A PATH TO INTEGRATION OF THE THEORY AND PRACTICE OF DEPRESSION: EVOLUTION, STRESS, AND PREDICTIVE PROCESSING

Valery Krupnik[*]
Department of Mental Health, Naval Hospital Camp Pendleton,
Camp Pendleton, CA, US

ABSTRACT

Depression has always been at center stage of psychiatry with many resources allocated and a significant progress made in its study and treatment. Still, it remains a wide-spread condition afflicting about 5-10% of the world population and is the leading cause of disability. Depression is a heterogeneous condition with multiple manifestations, symptoms, comorbidities, and degrees of severity compounding the challenge to its treatment. In this chapter, I suggest that progress in understanding the nature of depression and development of its general theory may assist

---

[*] Corresponding Author's Email: vkrupnik@gmail.com.

further advancements in its therapy. Evolutionary theory of depression has developed over several decades and is currently entrenched in the clinical thinking. More recently, a novel paradigm known as predictive coding (or predictive processing framework, PPF) has been proposed as a theoretical frame for understanding psychopathology including depression. PPF has been used as a conceptual bridge linking evolutionary and stress theories to explain mood/affective psychopathology. This emerging *Integrative Evolutionary-Stress response-PPF* (iESP) theory may offer useful insights for clinical practice. I review the rationale and recent developments in this integrative endeavor and discuss how the integrated perspective on depression can guide its treatment. To illustrate this with a clinical example, I present a novel evolutionary-based integrative therapy for depression.

Keywords: depression, predictive coding, free energy, allostasis, evolution, psychotherapy

1. INTRODUCTION

Many articles on depression start with the lamentation that depression is the cause of most disability time according to the world health organization's report (Ferrari et al. 2013). This is despite the long history of grappling with depression, which was described as early as the bible (1 Kings 19: 4-5, King James Version), and a large amount of resources both scientific and clinical allocated to study and treatment of this condition. Indeed, there are currently five classes of anti-depressant medications: tricyclic (TCAs) and related antidepressants; monoamine-oxidase inhibitors (MAOIs); selective serotonin re-uptake inhibitors (SSRIs); serotonin and noradrenaline reuptake inhibitors (SNRIs); and noradrenergic and specific serotonin antidepressants (NaSSAs). The total number of these medications is about thirty.

There are also about a couple of dozen psychotherapies for depression (Jorm et al. 2009). Several of them have obtained the evidence-based status, including Cognitive Behavioral, Interpersonal, Acceptance and Commitment, Mindfulness-Based Cognitive therapies. Together, they provide a sizeable arsenal for clinical practice. Still, major depression is the most frequently diagnosed mental disorder (Kessler et al. 2005, Rai et al. 2013), recurrence is the norm in depression (Solomon et al. 2000, Wakefield and Schmitz 2013), and over 20% of cases do not respond to conventional treatments (Fava 2003, Keller et al. 1992, Souery and Pitchot 2013). Moreover, as far as psychotherapy is concerned there is no clear treatment of choice (Shedler 2010) and more importantly, there has been no increase in the efficacy of therapies for depression in the last three decades (Cuijpers et al. 2019).

It appears that depressive disorders present a significant challenge that has not yet been well-understood let alone overcome. There can be a number of factors contributing to this challenge. One of them is lack of a unified *clinical-level* theory of depression. Depressive disorders are defined in the diagnostic manual DSM-5 (*Diagnostic and Statistical Manual of Mental Disorder,* 5th ed.; *DSM-5*; American Psychiatric Association, 2013) as a constellation of symptoms without tying them up to an etiology, as are most of the disorders in DSM-5. Theories of depression are many and they range from the neurochemical to social levels, constituting a matrix of overlapping theories that are yet to be integrated into a unified general theory (Bogdan, Nikolova, and Pizzagalli 2012).

The main symptom in depression is depressed mood, which is absence of mood and thus is a negative symptom, presenting another obstacle to treatment. Negative symptoms are more treatment resistant, as has been known for schizophrenia (Boonstra et al. 2012, Chang et al. 2011). Indeed, a negative symptom may stymie the therapist, because it represents a lack of target. It has been noted that depressed client's hopelessness may create a perception of ineffectiveness and a helpless feeling in the therapist, making sessions with depressed clients feel draining, suffused with the sense of helplessness on both sides, and empty (Berzoff and Hayes 1996). The prevalence of negative symptoms presents a challenge to talk therapy also due in part to the difficulty articulating the depressed state. In the incisive words of Lewis Wolpert, "Clinical depression is a strange state, and I have claimed that if you can describe your severe depression, you haven't truly experienced one" (Wolpert 2008, p. 2).

Depression is also known to have high comorbidity (Kessler et al. 1996) as well as diverse manifestations that may include agitation, high anxiety, hypersomnia (DSM-5), moreover, its different types such as melancholic vs non-melancholic may respond differentially to different kinds of therapy, e.g., anti-depressant medications vs CBT (Parker, Roy, and Eyers 2003).

Perhaps the most significant challenge to treating depression is that it is a systemic response of the whole organism, from the immune/inflammatory mechanisms to the hormonal/autonomic response, through alterations in emotion and cognition. Several recent reviews have highlighted the idea of depression as a systemic stress response, although from different theoretical perspectives (Badcock et al. 2017, Barrett, Quigley, and Hamilton 2016, Northoff et al. 2011).

In this chapter, I review theories of depression as a stress response, namely evolutionary and predictive coding theories, and suggest their integration that may serve as a *clinical-level* theory. I then discuss how such theory in conjunction with a theory of psychotherapy integration can guide therapy of depression. At the end, I give examples of psychotherapies guided by these theoretical considerations.

2. EVOLUTIONARY THEORY OF DEPRESSION

Being a meta-theory, evolutionary theory has the most explanatory power. Rather than explaining the mechanics of depression it seeks an explanation of the origin and purpose of the depressive process as a systemic response to environmental pressure. Addressing the ecology of organism's behavior, evolutionary theories seem best suited to provide a disorder-specific guidance to a therapist, since (a) ecology is the level, where clinical encounter occurs, and (b) evolutionary theories consider symptoms of depression not merely a constellation of the organism's reactions but a purposeful process, with which a therapy could be aligned. Evolutionary theory is a suitable clinical-level theory, since it does not only ask the mechanistic question *how* but the teleological *why*. The latter resonates with clinical encounter because it seeks to elucidate the meaning of what is happening to the patient. Uncovering that meaning has long been believed to have a therapeutic effect whether through insight, as in psychoanalysis/psychodynamic therapy (Freud 1966), change in core beliefs, as in cognitive therapy (Beck 1967), mindful awareness of the self, as in mindfulness-based therapies (Hayes, Strosahl, and Wilson 1999, Williams et al. 2007), or beliefs about others, as in interpersonal therapy (Klerman et al. 1984).

Evolutionary theory of depression is an umbrella term for a set of more specific theories considering depression an evolutionary conserved response to an inimical environment. Accordingly, these theories are largely based on animal models or analogs of depression. Regardless of the model, they all stipulate that depression evolved as a response to insurmountable adversity, i.e., an adversity that either cannot be overcome or where the cost of overcoming it is prohibitive.

Most notable of them are learned helplessness (Seligman 1972), based on the animal model where dogs develop depression-like symptoms in response to electric shocks they cannot escape; separation and loss, based on the model of infant monkeys separated from their mother (Bowlby 1980) and its modification called separation and grief and related to natural instances of infant's separation (Watt and Panksepp 2009); entrapment, based on the model of rodents restricted from free movement (Cryan, Mombereau, and Vassout 2005); defeat, based on the model of male rodents exposed to a bigger dominant male (Koolhaas et al. 1990). Other theories focus on such depressogenic conditions as loss of status, especially in adolescents (Gilbert 2000, Price et al. 1994), perceived loss of support as a trigger for postpartum depression (Hagen 1999). Some theorists conceptualize depression as a behavior meant to solicit social resources when the individuals believe they are unable to procure them themselves (Andrews and Durisko 2017).

I have proposed to conceptually integrate these models in one of *failure* and suggested an acronym FLED to represent them, standing for Failure: Loss, Entrapment, Defeat (Krupnik 2019b). Indeed, failure to meet one's needs is the underlying meaning of all the theorized etiologies of depression.

One of the loss models of particular interest in the context of this chapter was presented many decades ago and describes the behavior of a toddler pigtail monkey separated from its mother (Kaufman and Rosenblum 1967). The monkey at first becomes agitated and hyperactive seeking comfort with other maternal figures but once rejected it becomes passive and assumes a fetal posture. This represents a transition from protest to withdrawal. Such transition has been proposed as the core depressive reaction. "This sequence from protest to despair provides a powerful animal model of human clinical depression," (Zellner et al. 2011, p. 2). The authors consider it a prototype of such hallmark features of human depression as general resignation or 'giving up' comprising apathy, social withdrawal, and hopelessness. Even more importantly, after a while the monkey starts stimulating itself by exploring the environment and finds a companion toddler to play with. Such activity was considered by the model's authors the recovery stage of depression. In this view, depression is not a state of breakdown of the organism's functions but an adaptive process with its due course comprising a natural progression from protest to withdrawal and then to activation/recovery, a process that contains both the downward slide into depression and upward exit from it. Indeed, even untreated depressive episodes remit on average within twelve months (Furukawa, Kitamura, and Takahashi 2000, Spijker et al. 2002).

2.1. Depression as a Stress Response (DSR)

The diathesis model of pathology, which has a wide consensus in psychiatry, posits that psychopathology is a function of stress severity and innate vulnerability (Bleuler 1963, Robins and Block 1989). Depression, from the evolutionary standpoint, is an adaptive response to a stress that exceeds the organism's normative/optimal range of responses, making depression a particular kind of stress response, i.e., depressive stress response (DSR). Thus, a theory of stress provides a link between evolutionary theory of depression and its pathology.

Stress response is a universal property of self-organizing systems. Under destabilizing environmental pressure, they use the available resources to maintain their structure by minimizing the entropy and returning to stable states, of which they have a limited number (Mobus and Kalton 2015, Oken, Chamine, and Wakeland 2015). The idea of maintaining the organization and stability of internal environment was initially developed by C. Bernard and later captured in the concept of homeostasis (Cannon 1929). The idea of homeostasis is integral to the general theory of stress (Selye 1956), where the function of homeostasis is to return the organism to the baseline homeostatic state after having been perturbed by environmental stressors. The terms 'stress' and 'stressor' are sometimes defined differently in the literature. Here, I use 'stress' to mean an unstable condition of the organism caused by external stressors; 'stress response' then refers to the organism's re/actions directed at escaping stress by returning to a more stable homeostatic state. In living organisms (and supra-organismic systems such as ecosystems), stress response is a multilevel systemic process. It happens from the molecular level, e.g., mRNA taking alternative conformations (Ray et al. 2009) or protein aggregating (Tyedmers, Madariaga, and Lindquist 2008) under stress, to alterations in cognition (Ursin and Eriksen 2004).

A more recent update to the general theory of stress is the concept of allostasis (Sterling 2004, McEwen and Wingfield 2003). Allostasis literally means 'stability through change' and captures the idea that organisms constantly adjust their homeostatic state in order to maintain stability in the face of ever-changing environment. This process puts pressure on the organism called *allostatic load*. If the pressure exceeds the organism's capacity to cope, *allostatic overload* ensues. McEwen and Wingfield distinguish types 1 and 2 of allostatic overload (McEwen and Wingfield 2003). Type 1 refers to a situation, where the organism's energy resources are lower than its needs, in which case an emergency response is activated. Type 2 refers to a situation, where the organism has enough external resources but experiences a chronic allostatic load that gradually drives it into suboptimal homeostatic range. Both types can lead to pathology. An example of type 1 overload is a precipitous weight loss during famine, whereas type 2 overload can be exemplified by hypertension from cortisol imbalance in a situation of chronic psychological stress.

Elsewhere, I suggested that type 1 and 2 allostatic overloads correspond to "traumatic" and "pathogenic" stress responses, respectively (Krupnik 2018c). As an example, I drew a contrast between PTSD and depression. From the allostasis standpoint, evolutionary meaning of depressive stress response (DSR) is allostatic adaptation to failure (actual or perceived) of meeting one's needs, metabolic, psychological, and social. If so, DSR is expected to prepare the organism for the loss of resources and support. In such conditions, conservation of energy becomes most important, which can be achieved by disengaging from active life through emotional, cognitive, behavioral, and social withdrawal. This withdrawal is, indeed, a hallmark of the depressive phenotype.

There are multiple pathways leading to withdrawal in DSR. Thyroid hormones are essential for metabolism regulation and in particular for regulating energy expenditure vs conservation, such that hyperthyroidism leads to activation of metabolism and increase of the resting state energy expenditure and hypothyroidism having the opposite effect (Mullur, Liu, and Brent 2014). Notably, hypothyroidism causes anergia in humans, which is associated with symptoms of depression (Gold, Pottash, and Extein 1981), and subclinical hypothyroidism is a risk factor for depression (Tang et al. 2019). The fact that downregulation of metabolism by thyroid hormones has its depression-like corollary is in agreement with thyroid hormone role in preparing the organism for different life-history stages, for example, seasonal changes with the associated fluctuations in the resources availability. Thus, in hibernating ground squirrels, triiodothyronine levels are lowest at the stage of pre-hibernation and fattening (Wilsterman et al. 2015).

A central pathway to withdrawal, widely noted and researched in depression, is inhibition of the motivation/reward-seeking circuit. Inability to experience pleasure (anhedonia), loss of interest and motivation, and loss of appetite are ubiquitous symptoms of depression (DSM-5) and manifestations of dysregulated motivation and reward systems. The mesolimbic dopamine system comprising ventral tegmental area and nucleus accumbens is the main regulator of reward-seeking and motivation and has been implicated in mood regulation and depression-like behavior in rodents (Nestler and Carlezon 2006). The authors also note that hypothalamic neuropeptides regulating feeding behavior affect reward and mood regulation through the mesolimbic dopamine system, and manipulation of their receptors leads to either anti-depressant or depressogenic effects. This underscores the connection between depression and allostasis under resource-deficient conditions.

Childhood adversity has long been linked to increased risk of depression later in life (Kessler and Magee 2009). Recently, childhood material deprivation (food insecurity) but not emotional deprivation or trauma was linked to reward-seeking dysregulation in children and adolescents (Dennison et al. 2019). Noteworthy, the authors found that decreased integrity of the mesolimbic-frontal tract mediated the effect of material deprivation on depression, which confirms the central role of inhibition of the motivation circuit in DSR.

Depressed mood itself may be thought of as a representation of emotional withdrawal. Despite its widespread use both in scientific literature and common parlance the term 'depressed mood' is not easy to define. It does not have a clear neural correlate and is likely to be encoded by a multi-level distributed neural activity. Although depressed mood is often described in terms of such negative feelings as sadness, angst, despair, languor, wistfulness, etc., it is not reducible to any of them, since they can be experienced without depression. If we look at DSR as an allostatic transition to a state of low metabolic rate and motivation, depressed mood may be conceptualized as a generalized inhibition of positive emotional reactivity. I would also argue that at its deepest, depressed mood leads to inhibition of all emotional reactivity, i.e., to *functional affective blindness* except the meta-emotion of lack of feelings. Such meta-emotion is how depressed mood can be described. Defined this way, depressed mood appears crucial for recovery. Once emotional reactivity is inhibited or attenuated it helps the organism disengage from protesting the failure, preparing it for receptivity to available resources as opposed to seeking the unavailable ones (as in the above described orphaned pigtail monkey). Thus, depressed mood sets such a low emotional homeostatic set point, that previously ineffective sensory stimuli now rise above it and have a chance to jumpstart the motivation circuitry. The finding that behavioral activation therapy is effective for severe depression (Dimidjian et al. 2006) is consistent with this view, since any activity provides sensory stimulation both extero- and interoceptive. This conception of depressed mood is also consistent with evolutionary theory of the DSR arc: protest – withdrawal – recovery.

The evolutionary theory also helps explain the puzzle of contradictory manifestations of depression that include insomnia and hypersomnia, psychomotor retardation and agitation, loss of appetite and hyperphagia, apathy and anxiety (DSM-5). From the standpoint of the DSR arc, those symptoms are not contradictory but represent different DSR stages, where positive and negative symptoms are associated with the protest and withdrawal stages, respectively. It needs to be emphasized that DSR may not develop in a neatly linear fashion but more often is messy with back and forth vacillations between the stages and with mosaic of temporarily overlapping positive and negative symptoms. This has given rise to the notion of numerous types of depression (Blatt, D'Afflitti, and Quinlan 1976, Andrews and Durisko 2017), whereas from the evolutionary perspective those are but manifestations of DSR dynamics.

There has been an ongoing debate about the adaptive value of depression (Nesse 2000). One camp considers only symptoms of depression an adaption but clinical depression a maladaptive illness (Nesse 2000). Others argue that clinical depression can too be adaptive (Hagen 1999, Price et al. 1994, Watson and Andrews 2002). For example, Andrews and colleagues propose resource allocation hypothesis that regards clinically significant depressive symptoms including suicidal behavior as an evolved adaptation for adjusting resource allocation to environmental challenges (Andrews and Durisko 2017).

In the framework of DSR, the question of whether clinical depression is an adaptation or illness becomes about the degree of DSR optimization.

A well-optimized DSR is expected to efficiently progress through the arc from protest to recovery, whereas a poorly optimized one may get 'stuck' along the way. This suggests that some organisms may have a better optimized DSR than others and, therefore, susceptibility to depression should be, in part, hereditary. Indeed, major depression clearly has a genetic component (for a late review see McIntosh, Sullivan, and Lewis 2019).

Perhaps the main challenge to the adaptationist view of depression is its recurrent nature. A major depressive episode increases the probability of future episodes, where the future episodes appear to be triggered by less severe stressors. This observation led to kindling theory of depression's recurrence (Monroe and Harkness 2005). The authors suggest that a history of depression sensitizes the brain to stress, decreasing the threshold for consecutive episodes. There are data consistent with the kindling hypothesis, demonstrating changes following onset of depression, including hyper-reactivity of the HPA axis, more negative cognitive style, and personality change toward greater neuroticism (reviewed in (Monroe and Harkness 2005).

Recurrence of depression especially in light of sensitization to stress appears to refute its adaptive value, because higher susceptibility to illness compromises the organism's fitness. This argument, however, holds only if we consider depression an illness. From the DSR standpoint, sensitization to stress may represent a stress response memory akin to immune memory that shortens the response time to the challenge. Indeed, a large epidemiological study of the duration of depressive episodes has shown that a recurrent episode is, on average, two times shorter than a first (Spijker et al. 2002). Interestingly, in the same study, comorbid dysthymia increased the major depressive episode's duration almost twice. These findings may be interpreted as reflecting the adaptive value of 'kindling' DSR through creating a primed neuro-hormonal network for a prompt stress response, thus reducing the length of consecutive episodes. In this view, dysthymia represents malfunction of DSR, where it gets stuck between protest and withdrawal without moving to recovery. It is therefore expected that dysthymia would prolong the depressive episode.

The question of stress response optimization is essential for conceptualization of depression as illness as opposed to DSR. Where do we draw the line between an ecologically valid DSR and pathology? People with ecologically valid depression may and do end up in mental health clinics. Over-diagnosing depression appears to have become common (Parker 2007, Wakefield and Schmitz 2013). This, in turn, creates a dichotomy in defining mental health care as support vs treatment. Although it can be both, they nevertheless call for different approaches.

A stress response can be considered normative or pathological in reference to the level of the organism's functioning. In evolutionary view, an optimal stress response is one that maximizes the fitness *under the circumstances*. Accordingly, stress response should be regarded as a dynamic process, where the measure of its effectiveness is its outcome. For example, high fever during infection certainly decreases the organism's functioning, however, as long as it maximizes the chance for survival and minimizes the length of ailment it is adaptive. In the same way, the optimal range of DSR, as any other stress response, is context-dependent. It may differ significantly e.g., for someone coping with a loss of a relative among the rest of the surviving family compared to one who has lost a spouse without any remaining close relations. Decontextualized approach to mental disorders is a fallacy not particular to depression; elsewhere I argued that it concerns trauma-related disorders as well (Krupnik 2018c).

3. DEPRESSION AS A DISORDER OF FALSE INFERENCE: THE PREDICTIVE PROCESSING FRAMEWORK (PPF)

3.1. Psychopathology in PPF

A large body of research, described in numerous books and reviews, has accumulated about the mechanisms underlying the manifestations of depression. Since DSR is a systemic response, those mechanisms act at multiple levels, from the cognitive re-appraisal of self and the world through change in the activity of genes encoding cell factors (for recent reviews see e.g., (Ferrari and Villa 2017, Disner et al. 2011, Strain and Blumenfield 2018). These mechanistic descriptions do not by themselves establish an explanatory model of the processes that drive, organize, and coordinate DSR.

In the past two decades, a paradigm change generally called predictive coding or predictive processing framework (PPF) has transformed the fields of psychology and neuroscience including psychopathology (Clark 2013, Rao and Ballard 1999). PPF replaces the old paradigm of stimulus-processing-response with a different conception of brain functioning. According to it, brain constantly runs a *generative model* of the world, the self, and self-in-the-world. It is called generative because it continuously updates itself through the incoming sensory information. The model is *predictive* and *inferential* in that it predicts sensory sensations by *inferring* their causes. For example, as you have just read 'have', after seeing 'h' and 'v', your brain predicted the other letters, inferring the word 'have' from the context (on fast reading you would have most likely read 'have' in the misspelled version 'hve'). Sensory illusions are a common example of such inferential predictions (Hosoya, Baccus, and Meister 2005).

Through top-down efferent pathways, the generative model sends predictions that guide perception and action for the organism to regulate its internal environment and to meet its needs through negotiating the external one. In the process, it receives sensory information from the external world – through exteroception and the internal one – through interoception. When a sensory sensation differs from the prediction, this generates a *prediction error* (PE). PE is then passed bottom-up through afferent pathways to update the model in order to increase its accuracy. Computationally, PPF is a more powerful and efficient information processing than the unidirectional stimulus-processing-response one. In PPF, brain 'already knows' the world it is about to encounter and only needs the encounter to either confirm or update the knowledge instead of building it de novo (Huang and Rao 2011).

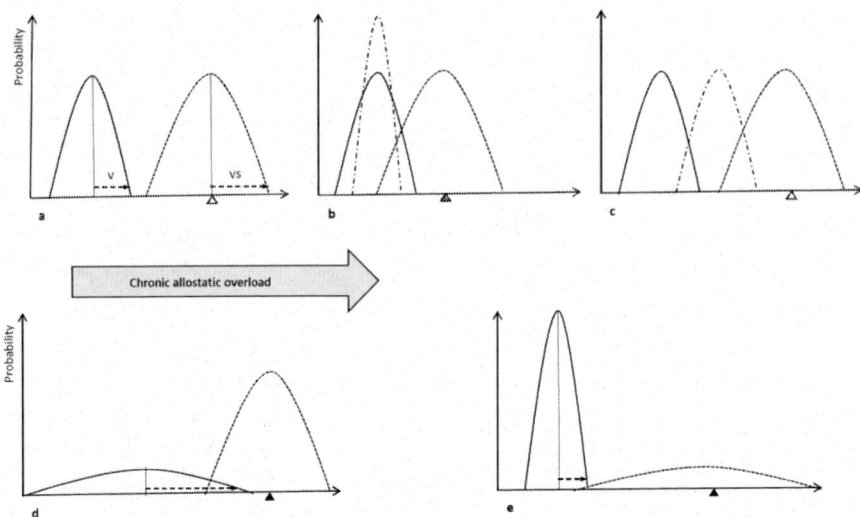

Figure 1. Generative model (GM) response to stress in Bayesian statistics.
───── prior, — · — posterior, ─ ─ ─ · sensory input, △ sensory input set point, ▲ sensory input set point by active inference, ▲ sensory input set point under allostatic overload.

a. GM with a distribution of prior with variance 'v' (precision=1/v) receives a sensory input with a variance 'vs' centered around a set point. The input generates prediction error (PE), thus creating stress.

b and c. Under normative stress, GM employs either of the following strategies to suppress PE:

b. GM resolves PE through active inference by adjusting the prior into a posterior of higher precision and selectively sampling the sensory information to confirm the posterior. Thus, it in effect creates a new distribution of the sensory input with a corresponding set point (a new subjective reality).

c. GM reacts by adjusting the prior into a posterior with a distribution overlapping the sensory input, thus suppressing the PE.

d and e. Under chronic stress, GM fails to resolve PE through either 'b' or 'c' strategies, thus creating a condition of chronic allostatic overload. It then uses either of the following strategies to suppress PE:

d. GM decreases the prior's precision, which increases the relative precision of PE (high expected PE precision) and makes it overweighted. This results in a self-inefficacious agnostic GM predicting the environment to be unpredictable.

e. GM increases the prior's precision, which decreases the relative precision of PE (low expected PE precision) and makes it underweighted. This results in a rigid GM insensitive to the environment, predicting it to be immutable with random fluctuations.

PF posits that brain uses Bayesian statistical *inference* to update its generative model (Friston, Kilner, and Harrison 2006). The Bayesian brain's predictions are represented by probability density functions called *priors* (the term is used interchangeably with *predictions, prior beliefs*, or just *beliefs*). Prior encodes the probability distribution of hypotheses (inferences) about the cause of a sensory event (in the above example the hypothesis was that the word 'have' was the cause you saw 'h' and 'v' in a close proximity). The event itself has a probability distribution called *likelihood*. Bayesian statistics establish a lawful relationship between a prior and the likelihood. Thus, prior encodes brain's prior learning. By encountering the likelihood (serving as evidence), which is a dynamic variable, the brain adjusts its prior into a *posterior* that becomes a new *empirical* prior, which represents the process of learning in Bayesian terms (Figure 1).

Although priors are probability density functions, in psychological literature they are, for simplicity's sake, often spoken about as beliefs. However, it must be underscored that in PPF, 'belief' is understood very broadly, ranging from a conscious verbalized thought to, for example, an unconscious expectancy of a visual contrast as in lateral retinal inhibition (Srinivasan et al. 1982) or expectancy of a neuronal firing rate. Priors are constantly tested by actual sensory stimuli, and mismatch generates PE that has to be resolved. This can be accomplished by either adjusting the initial prior into a posterior, that is through learning, (Figure 1) or adjusting the organism's behavior in such a way that the incoming stimuli match the prior. The latter process is called *active inference*. For exapmle, on fast reading your visual cortex might not have 'noticed' the misspelled 'example' in an act of active inference, where you have chosen to read words not the letters. Alternatively, your priors might have adjusted to allow for misspelled words in a published product despite the power of spellcheck.

It makes sense that brain's generative model would strive to resolve PE for the sake of its accuracy. After all, it evolved to enable the organism to know what to expect from the environment in order to respond to it in the most adaptive way. However, what, if anything, is the guiding principle organizing the super-complex brain activity in its drive for accuracy?

More recently, PPF has been 'high-powered' by the free-energy idea, which has been suggested as such principle (Friston 2010). The free-energy law suggests that an essential property of any adaptive self-organizing system (of which brain is one) is minimization of its *variational free energy*. Variational free energy is an informatics term referring to the upper boundary on surprisal or *uncertainty* about the state of the system. Minimization of free energy thus leads to decreased uncertainty. This principle is related to Ashby's principle of self-organization, where self-organizing dynamical systems always evolve toward reducing their statistical entropy, i.e., uncertainty about their state (Ashby 1947). Both are related to the second law of thermodynamics stating that in natural processes, entropy always increases, implying that self-organization can be viewed as a process of entropy minimization. Accordingly, brain is seen as a system that is constantly evolving toward minimization of the variational free energy of the generative model it embodies, thus reducing the uncertainty (statistical entropy) about its sensory states. Brain accomplishes that through iterative cycles of resolving PE (Figure 2) by either posterior learning or active inference. In this view, *all* brain activity serves minimization of its free energy, which is why the free-energy principle has been proposed as a unifying theory of brain (Friston 2010).

Free energy minimization happens in the brain through hierarchical information passaging (Friston, Kilner, and Harrison 2006), where high level multi-modal integrated representations in association cortex transmit predictions down to sensory and motor networks, while sensory input is transmitted back up to the association cortex (Figure 2). Prediction error estimating units then compute PE by comparing prediction to the sensory input. Deep layer pyramidal cortical neurons are believed to transmit top-down predictions and superficial layer pyramidal neurons - the bottom-up sensory information (Friston, Kilner, and Harrison 2006).

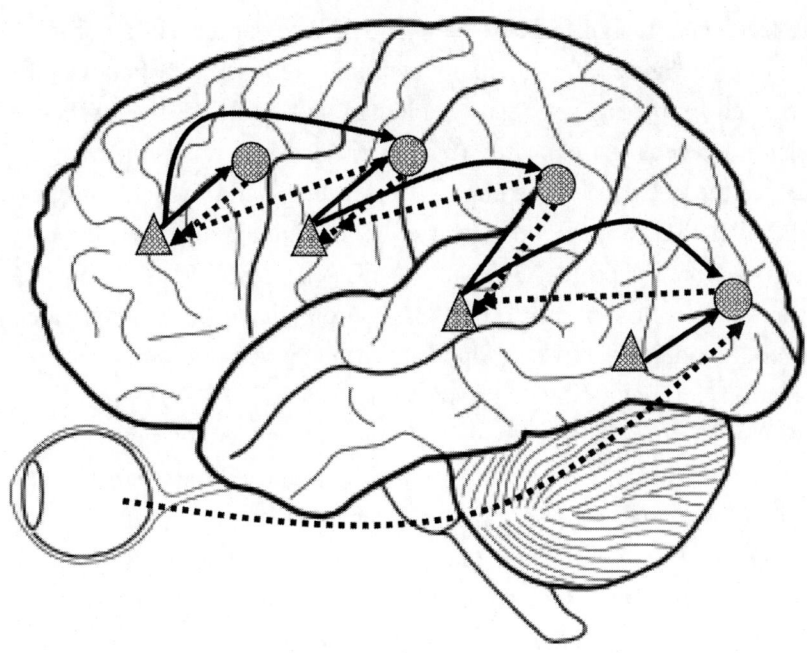

Figure 2. Hierarchical message passaging in predictive processing.
⬤ error unit, ▲ prediction unit, ▬▬ backward prediction signaling, ▬ ▬ forward prediction error signaling.
Generative circuits encoding representations send top-down predictions to primary sensory areas, while sensory information encoding circuits signal bottom-up to higher general domain representation areas. Mismatch between prediction and sensory information generates prediction error. The generative model suppresses prediction error either by adjusting predictions or by manipulating the sensory input through active inference.

One of the central tasks of brain's generative model is to compute the relative importance of PE vs the prediction. Real world is inherently dynamic and 'noisy,' and brain has to have a way to filter the noise out, otherwise the stability of its generative model may be undermined. The process of estimating the importance of PE relative to the prediction is called *precision weighting* (Feldman and Friston 2010). The term 'precision weighting' is more often applied to PE. Here, however, I apply it equally to PE and predictions for a greater conceptual clarity given the clinical importance of their reciprocal relationship explored in the following sections.

Precision of a signal is defined as the inverse variance of its probability distribution (Figure 1), which, in neuronal networks, is believed to be determined by the synaptic gain (Feldman and Friston 2010). When PE's precision exceeds the expected (by the prediction's precision) range, that increases the network's free energy (uncertainty) and triggers suppression of the PE. Precision is believed to be modulated by 'out-of-network' neurons. Norepinephrine- (Peters, McEwen, and Friston 2017) and dopaminergic (Friston et al. 2012) neurons have been implicated in precision modulation, which appears fitting given their central role in motivation and attention. In psychology, precision is cognate to the concept of stimulus salience which is largely dependent on both.

If we consider the free-energy principle a unified theory of brain, then malfunction of predictive coding should be considered a unified theory of psychopathology. Indeed, in the last decade, there has been an avalanche of studies framing psychiatric disorders as aberrant predictive coding. Examples include psychosis (Powers, Mathys, and Corlett 2017), depression (Badcock et al. 2017, Barrett, Quigley, and Hamilton 2016), disorders of personality (Moutoussis et al. 2014), ADHD (Dołęga 2018), autism (Lawson, Rees, and Friston 2014), PTSD (Wilkinson, Dodgson, and Meares 2017), functional neurological disorders (Edwards et al. 2012). In all cases, dysfunctional precision weighting has been implicated in their etiology.

Theory of homeostasis and in particular its allostasis development has recently been integrated with PPF (Sterling 2004, Peters, McEwen, and Friston 2017). This integration is based on three main premises. One concerns the function of allostasis in the organism's adaptation to changing environment. For such an adaptation to be most efficient, the organism should not just react to the change but anticipate it (Sterling 2004). An anticipatory response may have several advantages including a) shorter reaction time, since the organism is already in a 'standby' status, b) a better coordinated response, because anticipation can be a centrally controlled systemic state, and c) an anticipatory state may encode a range of expected reactions thus safeguarding against over-reaction to random fluctuations in the environment and supporting the system's stability.

The second premise, related to the first, concerns *how* the organism can anticipate change. For that, PPF provides a heuristic means. Brain's generative model constantly predicts the future while being updated by the present. In particular, the model includes expectations about the range of environmental fluctuations (both in internal and external environment), and when the range is exceeded, the model recalibrates itself adjusting its priors into posteriors (Figure 1) and engages via active inference behavioral and physiological strategies matching the fluctuations. This is the suggested mechanism of stress response (Sterling 2004, Peters, McEwen, and Friston 2017). Should the strategies be successful in mitigating the environmental impact, the organism returns to its homeostatic state, otherwise (if allostatic overload arises), it undergoes allostatic transition to a different, usually less adaptive homeostatic state. Elsewhere (Krupnik 2018c), I defined the former outcome as normative stress response and the latter as pathogenic stress response.

The third premise links the first two. It provides a guiding and organizing principle for brain generative model's response to stress, which is the above mentioned free-energy principle. In view of this principle, stress equals uncertainty (Peters, McEwen, and Friston 2017), because stress arises when the environmental challenge exceeds the predicted range, thereby increasing the model's free-energy/uncertainty. Since brain's universal function, according to the principle, is to minimize its uncertainty, it attempts to do so through active inference or, if it proves ineffective, through re-adjusting its generative model to a new set point ('new normal'). For example, under chronic psychosocial stress, an organism may develop hypertension as a new tonic set point (McEwen and Wingfield 2003) to keep the blood flow ready for the expected phasic response to an environmental challenge.

3.2. Depression as a Disorder of Precision Weighting

In the *Integrative Evolutionary-Stress response-PPF* (iESP) view of psychopathology, depression emerges as a disorder of arrested stress response stuck at the pathogenic stress response stage, such that the allostatic overload persists even after the external challenge ceases. PPF application to depression has, in recent years, cropped up in the literature. Badcock and colleagues developed evolutionary systems theory to address the development of depressive phenotype and its adaptive function. They propose that depression evolved as an adaptation for resolving the uncertainty of social challenges (Badcock et al. 2017). In an adverse social environment, the brain goes into depressed mode by overweighting the precision of social prediction errors (PE), making the person more sensitive to aversive social cues while decreasing confidence in his social predictions. This mode is supposed to facilitate learning (building a posterior set of priors) about the causes of social cues. However, if the depressed mode perseveres, it can lead to an aberrant generative model with a high-precision negative bias. In that case, active inference can produce a set of behaviors and physiological responses confirming the bias, e.g., social withdrawal, avoidance of reward-seeking and exploration, anhedonia, loss of appetite, etc., leading to a self-perpetuating depressive cycle of clinical depression.

Other work emphasizes high-level cognitive priors that create a negative bias in Bayesian inferences about self and others in the depressed mind. Such priors form core beliefs that exert top-down control over the generative model and are fulfilled through active inference, which then results in second-order empirical priors, that is, predictions about efficacy (or rather inefficacy, in case of depressive generative model) of one's action (Moutoussis et al. 2014). The more empirical priors confirm the first-order core beliefs, the greater becomes their precision, reinforcing the model's negative bias.

There also has been emphasis on the role of interoception in depressive stress response (DSR) and allostasis (Paulus and Stein 2010, Barrett, Quigley, and Hamilton 2016, Seth and Friston 2016), where depression is regarded as a consequence of dyshomeostasis or, in other words, "a disorder of allostasis." The cause of dyshomeostasis is seen in inefficient predictive coding, in particular, predictive coding of the internal model of metabolic and physiological functions. Interoception is the gateway for sensory information about body states to the brain. Under stress, the internal model sends descending interoceptive predictions about the expected change in the body to prepare it for an appropriate response to the stressor, e.g., increased heart and breathing rates in face of danger to prepare for a quick escape. Likewise, in the absence of danger, the model will predict the baseline heart and breathing rates. However, interoceptive signals always have natural fluctuations and are, in this sense, 'noisy.' An efficient internal model filters the noise out by predicting a certain threshold for PEs' precision, above which they can affect the priors.

Chronic stress is known to present high risk for depression (McGonagle and Kessler 1990). Under chronic stress, e.g., when an organism is trapped in a toxic (or perceived as toxic) environment, interoceptive PE may become underweighted through the negative feedback loop, since the priors are "locked in" predicting stress response (Barrett, Quigley, and Hamilton 2016). The more they are underweighted, the more precise will the 'stress' priors become, underweighting the errors even further, thus touching off a depressive downward spiral.

In order to integrate these lines of reasoning I suggest a model of depression as a disorder of precision weighting as illustrated in Figure 3. The model integrates the ideas of dysregulated intero- and exteroceptive precision weighting. In it, a brain's generative model faced with an inescapable adversity starts overweighting exteroceptive prediction errors due to ineffectiveness of its (hedonic) priors[1] in resolving PE through either learning or active inference, which would lead to persisting allostatic overload (high uncertainty = stress, Peters, McEwen, and Friston 2017). In such circumstance, decreasing precision of the priors relative to the errors (Figure 1) is the only option for suppressing PE and decreasing the uncertainty (free energy), i.e., low precision of expectation means low discrepancy with the incoming sensory information and, therefore, suppression of PE. If you are walking in a dense fog and trip over a stump you did not spot in time, you would not be as surprised as you would tripping over it in a crisp clear air.

---

[1] Hedonic prior is a prediction about pleasurable/noxious effect of external events, e.g., social encounters.

The low prior/high PE precision of exteroception strategy has its limitation, because it leaves the generative model in a world of inherent unpredictability and, therefore, in a state of uncertainty above its set point. In order to compensate for it, the generative model underweights interoceptive errors while increasing the precision of interoceptive (allostasis) priors[2] (Figure 3). This will also lead to decreased free energy but through an inverse mechanism, i.e., suppressing interoceptive PE by underweighting their precision. As a result, depressive generative model is 'locked in' two pathogenic cycles feeding into each other (Figure 3). The exteroceptive, where negative sensory input becomes overweighted, making predictions about the environment imprecise, which may subjectively feel as overwhelming. The interoceptive, where this imprecision is matched (compensated for) by interoceptive (allostasis) priors and underweighted interoceptive errors, thus creating a physiologically/metabolically embodied mirror model of the overwhelming (noxious) environment. Emergence of this model may be seen as an act of active physiological inference, fulfilling the low precision of exteroceptive priors. Such extero/interoceptive dynamics may serve as a mental representation of unmanageable stress.

This model needs at least two extensions. One is to explain how stress could touch off the described cycles. Second is to place the model in a dynamic context in order to accommodate the idea of depressive stress response as a *process* not just a state.

In order to explain how the hypothesized dysregulation of precision weighting is brought about in depression, we may invoke the above mentioned concept of *failure* (FLED) and its central role (according to evolutionary theory) in depression. As a mental representation, failure is best defined as self-efficacy or rather its inversion – self-inefficacy. Self-efficacy is a concept referring to people's expectations of their ability to successfully execute actions toward a desirable outcome (Bandura 1977).

---

[2] Allostasis prior is a prediction about physiological reactions to stress, e.g., levels of HPA hormones or heart rate.

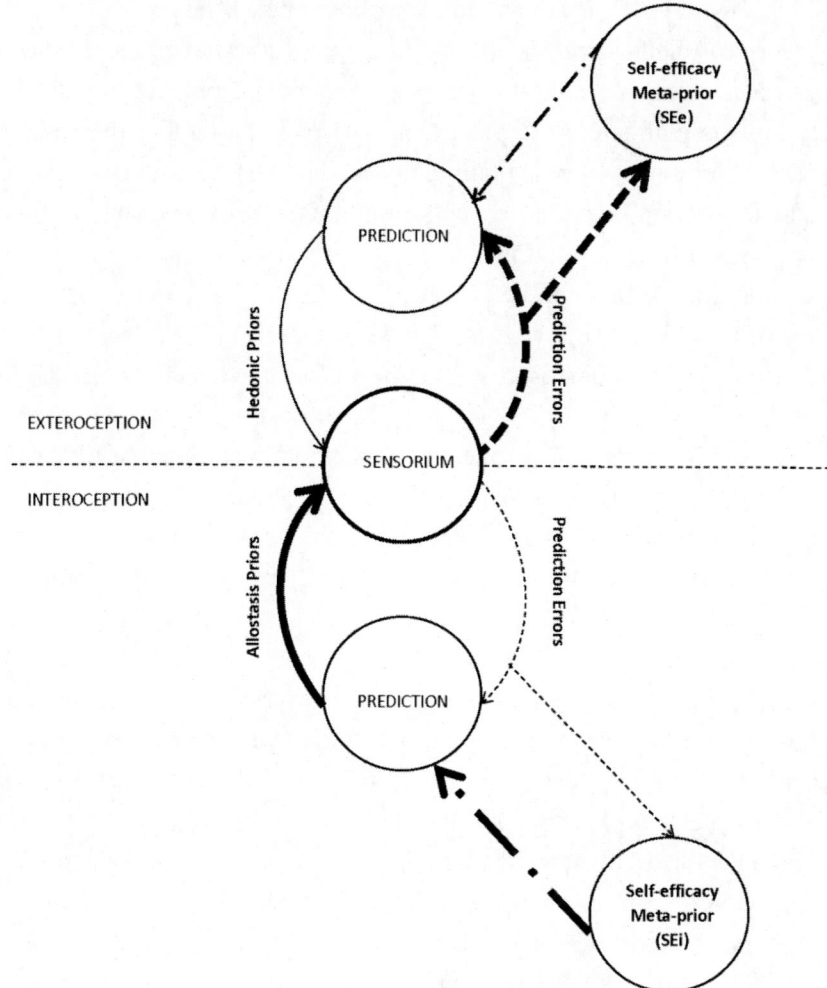

Figure 3. Precision weighting in depressive stress response (DSR).
On the exteroceptive side, chronic failure to meet one's (hedonic) needs leads to decrease of the precision of hedonic priors, while exteroceptive prediction errors become overweigted. This is facilitated by decrease of the self-efficacy meta-prior's precision, which is, in turn, driven by overweigted prediction errors.
On the interoceptive side, chronic failure leads to allostatic overload driving the increase of allostatsis priors' precision, while underweighting prediction errors. Thereby, the depressed brain is 'locked in' dysregulated precision weighting that creates the perception of exhausted, relatively insensitive body trapped in an unpredictable inimical world.
────── priors, ─ · ─ · · meta-priors, ─ ─ ─ ─ ─ prediction errors.

In PPF terms, self-efficacy is a prediction about one's efficacy. In line with the theory of self-efficacy, allostatic self-efficacy has recently been suggested as a high-level metacognitive prediction about the organism's ability to cope with stress (Stephan et al. 2016). In particular, the authors suggest that prolonged stress entailing dyshomeostasis leads to decrease of self-efficacy, which is caused by persisting unresolved interoceptive PEs. In turn, low self-efficacy is fulfilled by active inference through avoiding active coping as in 'learned helplessness' (Seligman 1972) and sustained by overweighted interoceptive PEs. This may create another self-sustaining depressive cycle: dyshomeostasis – low self-efficacy - dyshomeostasis. In accord with this theory, I suggest that self-efficacy serves as a master regulator of precision weighting in the extero/interoceptive balance. Specifically, it sends top-down predictions about precision of the organism's lower-level predictions about exteroceptive sensory information (Figure 3). High self-efficacy predicts high-precision exteroceptive priors that resolve/suppress prediction errors (of a relatively low-precision) through active inference (proactive coping behaviors), whereas *self-inefficacy* predicts low-precision priors that are 'permissive' to prediction errors, resolving them by further decreasing the priors' precision and fulfilling the self-inefficacy prediction through inaction as in 'learned helplessness.' This idea has been aptly expressed in a recent conceptualization of depressed mood in PPF, "major depression occurs when the brain is certain that it will encounter an uncertain environment, i.e., the world is inherently volatile, capricious, unpredictable and uncontrollable" (Clark, Watson, and Friston 2018, p 2278). Chronic unpredictable stress is a widely used animal model of depression (Katz 1982).

The hypothesized role of self-efficacy in depression ultimately raises the question of how FLED may effect the efficacy-to-inefficacy transition. I find the key to this question in the above discussed concept of depression as a dynamic (protest-withdrawal-recovery) process as opposed to a state. At the initial, *protest*, stage of DSR, the brain's exteroceptive priors attempt to resolve noxious sensory information coming from the toxic environment by active inference through initiating coping behaviors, e.g., escape, avoidance, confrontation, problem solving, etc. This reaction fulfills the self-efficacy prediction of competency and increases the precision of predicted favorable outcome. Interoceptive allostasis priors react accordingly by increased precision to accommodate the anticipated metabolic/physiological stress-associated demands, e.g., increased heart rate, blood pressure, glucose metabolism, HPA upregulation, etc. If the desirable outcome is reached, the organism returns to its homeostatic state, its self-efficacy predictions grow more precise, the stress response is learned and can be deployed next time with even greater effectiveness.

If the organism *fails* to reach the desired outcome, an inversion of the above process is likely: the exteroceptive PEs fail to resolve, and the high level of free energy 'forces' a decrease of the exteroceptive priors' precision to 'accommodate' the PE (Figure 1). This, in turn, drives down the precision of self-efficacy turning it into self-inefficacy, which further 'relaxes' the exteroceptive priors' precision. Interoceptive priors then grow ever more rigid predicting a higher level of metabolic/physiological stress, even if the initial external stressors relent, thus underweighting interoceptive PEs, i.e., making the organism relatively insensitive to interoceptive stimuli. Such inversion represents the *withdrawal* stage of DSR. At its most extreme, self-inefficacy may lead to a paradoxical state of complete inaction, to the point of catatonia, while in a state of acute stress, as in catatonic depression (Moskowitz 2004). Of note, Moscowitz considers catatonia an ancient evolutionary adaptation related to *freeze response* and meant to prevent triggering predators' attack reaction to the prey's movement. Interestingly, a recent account of functional paralysis conceptualizes it as an act of active inference to fulfill the hyper-precise prediction of the patient's motor inefficacy (Edwards et al. 2012). If we generalize this idea to the global systemic inefficacy, it will fit the described model of DSR's withdrawal stage.

The next and final stage of DSR is *recovery*. What could possibly help a brain out of the trap of being 'locked in' between a hyper-precise self-inefficacy and hyper-precise interoceptive predictions of stress (Figure 3)? I suggest that another inversion of the precision weighting dynamic, this time from bottom up, may occur after the withdrawal stage. It starts at the level of interoception. Remember, that both interoceptive predictions and sensations are probability distributions and as such have random fluctuations within their respective ranges (Figure 1). Once withdrawal is completed or 'hit the bottom,' the mean of interoceptive priors' distribution stops moving in the direction of predicting high stress and settles around a new 'set point,' which becomes the new interoceptive normal. This increases the probability that an interoceptive prediction 'falls' on the positive (lower stress) side of the norm, i.e., less bad is perceived as good. If such a prediction is matched by a low-stress interoceptive sensation (they also fluctuate around a set point) its frequency will increase 'pulling' the tail of prior distribution toward a lower-stress posterior, while decreasing its precision. Given such dynamics, a stream of pleasurable/low-stress interoceptive stimuli would create a recovery momentum, where the priors' precision will further decrease, resulting in increased PE precision weighting. For recovery to proceed, such momentum has to be reinforced by the corresponding dynamic of the self-efficacy meta-prior (Figure 3). The same logic of 'new normal' applies here. Once withdrawal reaches its completion, and self-efficacy hits the bottom, it becomes insensitive to further failure and settles around a low mean/set point. Then, any random act of successfully exercising one's agency could generate an upward self-efficacy momentum that would uphold such momentum in exteroceptive priors, which, in turn, would feed into the increasing weighting of interoceptive PE and 'relaxing' of interoceptive priors. Once that happens, the whole DSR cycle will start in reverse: increased self-efficacy will increase predictions of positive interoceptive sensations and behavioral outcomes, whose probability will be relatively high, because the whole system starts from a low set point.

The above discussion about the role of self-efficacy meta-prior in DSR only concerned self-efficacy in relation to the external world (SEe). Self-efficacy, however, can also be defined in relation to the internal environment (SEi) as "allostatic self-efficacy" (Stephan et al., 2016), which is understood as the organism's ability to accommodate allostatic load (or in simpler terms, adapt to stress). In the PPF model of DSR (Fig 3), SEi represents a mirror image of SEe, and its role in DSR can be described following the same logic. That is, during the protest stage, SEi's precision grows (to accommodate the allostatic overload resulted from failure and breakdown of SEe), which drives the increase of allostasis priors' precision (Figure 3). As DSR comes to its withdrawal stage, this dynamic reaches its peak, making the SEi susceptible to reversal of its cycle (as discussed above for SEe), opening a path to recovery. To paraphrase Clark et al. (Clark, Watson, and Friston 2018, p 2278) we may say that depression happens when certain in its failure organism is internally prepared for the failure's consequences.

Whether SEe and SEi can directly regulate each other remains an open question that, to my knowledge, has yet to be empirically addressed. Given the brain's functional redundancy such direct regulatory loop appears likely although not necessary. The indirect regulatory loop (Fig 3) may suffice.

One might ask, what about the failure? It is still there and should, according to the proposed model, pull the organism back into depression. This is the most important point of the iESP model of depression. Failure that has already happened and brought the DSR to completion of the withdrawal stage is, in a sense, not a failure any longer. It becomes included in the posterior distribution of the organism's predictions about its self-efficacy and outcomes of its interactions with the environment. Hence, it does not generate a prediction error and bias the mean of that distribution anymore, making the organism relatively insensitive to it. That failure, one could say, has been mentally 'metabolized.' An accepted failure is a failure overcome.

We could use a pendulum analogy to describe the above explicated DSR dynamics. If there is a force systematically biasing a pendulum to the left, it will move more and more in this direction with every swing. Once it reaches as far left as it can, it will swing as much left as it will right around the new set point. After that, should there be any momentum to the right; the pendulum will start moving right with every swing, following that momentum (also see Figure 1 for comparison). As the organism settles into a self-inefficacy prediction, any random sensory stimulation that does not confirm it (could be as simple as a friendly smile) has the potential of creating such rightward momentum. What if such a momentum fails to either emerge or carry the organism to recovery? In that case, depression can be lethal, which may also be considered an adaptation meant to eliminate excessively vulnerable to depression individuals and their genomes from the population (Syme, Garfield, and Hagen 2016). Such individuals could be a burden on the population's resources (both social and material) and decrease the fitness of its gene pool.

An interesting corollary to the iESP model of depression is that which helps the brain out of depression makes it vulnerable to its recurrence. Once a failure becomes encoded in the brain's distribution of priors it carries certain vulnerabilities. One is associated with the potential for the organism to fulfill such a prior through active inference, which has a chance to touch off another DSR. Also, should another failure of the kind occur, its perception will be shaped by the encoded 'failure' priors including the one of self-inefficacy, which is likely to speed up DSR progression. The idea that DSR may be accelerated in a recurrent depressive episode is supported by the finding that a recurrent episode is on average twice as short as the initial one (Spijker et al. 2002). These considerations would explain the 'kindling' hypothesis of depression's recurrence (Monroe and Harkness 2005).

It is important to emphasize that the described model is a significant simplification. The mentioned predictions and sensory information are multi-domain and multi-level processes. Even within interoception there are multiple domains including breathing, cardio-vascular, nociceptive, gastro-intestinal, each of them under both neural and humoral control. Self-efficacy is also multi-domain and multi-level from one's belief about winning a tennis match to his belief about controlling his bladder. Such complexity in combination with the complex dynamics of DSR can account for multiple manifestations and types of depression. Noteworthy, DSR's dynamics can explain many of the apparent inconsistencies. For example, depressive symptoms may include anxiety and apathy, insomnia and hypersomnia, agitation and immobility. If we allow that the hyperarousal symptoms of anxiety, agitation, and insomnia are manifestations of the protest stage, whereas the hypo-arousal ones – of the withdrawal stage, there will be no contradiction. In the same way, we can reconcile the notion of "high interoceptive surprise" in depression (Stephan et al. 2016) with "relative insensitivity to prediction errors" (Barrett, Quigley, and Hamilton 2016). Again, the former is likely to associate with the protest stage and the latter – the withdrawal one.

Another simplification is presenting DSR as a linear protest-withdrawal-recovery progression. The linear progression is but one possibility; others include cycling from protest to withdrawal and back, from partial recovery to withdrawal, or being stuck halfway at any of the stages. As all complex dynamic systems do (Barton 1994), brain's generative model may have a number of quasi stable states (attractors) where it can be 'stuck' for a length of time. The complexity of DSR dynamics can explain why it can take so long – on average twelve months (Furukawa, Kitamura, and Takahashi 2000, Spijker et al. 2002) - for a depressive episode to spontaneously remit. For a positive momentum to emerge internaly-directed self-efficacy (SEi) and interoceptive priors should reach their peak at about the same time as externaly-directed self-efficacy (SEe) and exteroceptive priors 'bottom out' (Figure 3), which is not a given due to their multi-domain and multi-level nature as well as a relative autonomy from each other.

It may be helpful to illustrate what the model may look like in clinical psychological language, especially that it is meant, as was mentioned from the outset, to be a *clinical-level* theory. Bereavement and grief may be considered a benign case of depression, moreover, grief is believed to follow similar to DSR psychodynamics (Kübler-Ross 1997), where denial, anger, and bargaining are akin to the protest stage, and acceptance – to withdrawal. Loss of a loved one constitutes a failure to meet one's relational needs. Bereavement is understood here in a broad sense as inaccessibility of the object of love/attachment for various reasons, not necessarily death. Such inaccessibility generates a flood of hedonic prediction errors coming from external stimuli signaling the absence of the object, i.e., lack of physical presence, lack of communication, absence from expected future events. The usual first reaction to bereavement is protest, where the mind attempts to suppress the PEs by either underweighting them (denial) or through active inference such as acting out, e.g., frequent visits to the grave, talking to or stalking the object, or even hallucinating them (Grimby 1993). Affective manifestations include anxiety, agitation, anger.

Futility of these attempts creates a meta-prediction error that is resolved through posterior learning of failure in the form of self-inefficacy meta-prior or low SEe precision (Figure 3). Such SEe prior is then matched by decrease in precision of the lower level hedonic beliefs about the object of love (acceptance of loss, loss of hope, mental distancing), which is associated with overweighted exteroceptive PEs, which brings the mind to the stage of withdrawal/resignation. Affective manifestations include apathy, sadness, angst.

In parallel, interoceptive predictions of stress increase in precision in order to prepare the organism for allostasis to the new environment bereft of the object of love and, therefore, inhospitable. This process is bootsrapped by increased precision of SEi predicting readiness for allostatic overload. It leads to underweighted interoceptive PEs, resulting in a chronic state of stress with its physiological corollary of fatigue, loss of appetite and often weight, loss of interest, motivation, and pleasure, decreased libido, downregulation of the adaptive immune system (Barrett, Quigley, and Hamilton 2016). This creates selective interoceptive blindness to all sensations but ones that fulfill the stress predictions, thus 'locking the mind in' between low-precision SEe and high-precision SEi.

Once self-inefficacy sets in, and prior beliefs about the object of love lose their precision, the loss is accepted. This acceptance then becomes part of the posterior beliefs, which then accommodate prediction errors associated with the loss (Figure 1). The act of accepting itself effects change, thereby generating a prediction error contradicting the self-inefficacy prior, thus increasing the chance for its reversal. Such reversal will then 'rescue' exteroceptive priors, in turn, 'relaxing' the pressure on interoceptive stress priors creating momentum for a further reversal of the 'lock-in' dynamics and, therefore, for recovery. The likelihood of such reversal increases with exteroceptive sensations fulfilling SEe priors such as sense of competence, goal attainment, reward gain, as well as with pleasurable interoceptive sensations generating an error contradicting the allostasis priors (Figure 3). In other words, resumption of active productive life will carry the momentum on.

The presented iESP model is highly speculative; it needs to be mathematically formalized and empirically tested. There is a large volume of empirical evidence compatible with it that has been comprehensively reviewed. Association of depression with allostatic adaptation has been noted in evolutionary system theory (Badcock et al. 2017) it has also led to the notion of depressive phenotypes (Andrews and Durisko 2017). Both reviews summarize the evidence for depression as an adaptation to complex social challenges. Evidence for the role of interoception in allostasis as it applies to depression has been the subject of a number of recent reviews (e.g., Seth and Friston 2016, Barrett, Quigley, and Hamilton 2016, Peters, McEwen, and Friston 2017). Finally, the role of self-efficacy as a meta-prior in depression has also been discussed (Stephan et al. 2016, Paulus and Stein 2010, Clark, Watson, and Friston 2018). In an animal model of spontaneous recovery from depression, one of the most salient neural markers of recovery was restoration of normal functional connectivity between somatosensory and frontal cortices, which underscores the central role of mutual regulation between higher order representations and interoception in DSR dynamics (Khalid et al. 2016).

Here, I want to highlight the major predictions of iESP account of DSR. One is that self-efficacy decreases in parallel with decrease of interoceptive sensitivity, as depression progresses from protest to withdrawal. More importantly, they are predicted to affect each other through a feedback loop (Figure 3). It has, indeed, been demonstrated that depressive and anxiety symptoms tend to associate with decreased and increased interoceptive awareness, respectively (Pollatos, Traut-Mattausch, and Schandry 2009), which fits the idea that the protest and withdrawal stages of DSR are qualitatively different psycho-physiological states, and that the concept of depression as a process rather than a state more accurately reflect its nature.

Another prediction is that spontaneous recovery from depression is most likely when both interoceptive sensitivity and self-efficacy have bottomed out. In this state, a positive momentum in one would be supported by such a momentum in the other (Figure 3). This hypothesis, while challenging to be tested in humans, may be readily explored in animal models of spontaneous recovery such as used by Khalid et al. (Khalid et al. 2016). Related to this hypothesis is the prediction that depressive episodes with mixed presentation, i.e., anxious and agitated depression, may take longer to remit. It has long been observed that a comorbid anxiety disorder is a risk factor for prolonged depression (Clayton et al. 1991, Brown et al. 1996). A more recent observation indicates that a history or subthreshold symptoms of depression are a risk factor for both depressive and anxiety disorders, whereas a history and subthreshold symptoms of anxiety predicts anxiety disorders only (Karsten et al. 2018). This is consistent with the view of DSR progression from protest (associated with anxiety) to withdrawal. Therefore, anxiety symptoms alone may be insufficient to prime for DSR, because, I suggest, they lack the self-inefficacy experience, central to the withdrawal stage. In general, all mood, affective, and trauma-related disorders can be conceptualized within iESP. For example, from the Bayesian brain standpoint, the adaptive function of negative emotion is to signal an error in predicting the sensory sensation in order to stimulate inferential learning about its cause; such learning will then resolve the prediction error and decrease the free energy, thus downregulating the emotion (Joffily and Coricelli 2013). Consequently, false inference would lead to emotion dysregulation. Analysis of other disorders is, however, beyond this chapter's scope.

4. iESP-Informed Treatment of Depression: Strategic Modification of Priors (SMOP)

There are two main premises that iESP offers for guiding treatment of depression. One is that depression is an arrested depressive stress response (DSR); the other is that such arrest is due to the brain 'locked in' an aberrant precision weighting (Figure 3). These premises point at two respective targets for therapeutic intervention: the developmental course of DSR and precision weighting.

4.1. The Developmental Course of DSR as a Target for Intervention

Evolutionary theory of depression has been in clinical discourse for nearly half a century. To my knowledge, only two psychotherapies have made explicit use of it. One is evolutionary-driven cognitive therapy for depression (Giosan et al. 2014). Its approach is to identify threats to the patient's fitness and target them with cognitive-behavioral methods, which is achieved through cognitive restructuring of the mismatch between evolutionary-driven beliefs about one's fitness and a more adaptive reality-based understanding of one's opportunities and limitations. It also employs behavioral modification targeting the fitness-compromising behaviors.

The other therapy is called Treating Depression Downhill (TDD), whose approach is different in that in its initial phases it seeks to facilitate the DSR by helping it 'bottom out' through the transition from protest to withdrawal (Krupnik 2014). Such transition is aided by fostering the experience of acceptance rather than targeting cognitive biases or behavioral modification. TDD is the only therapy that explicitly helps depression to *progress down*. In that, it follows the iESP's contention that a) this progression is the function of DSR, and b) that recovery is more likely from DSR's 'bottom.'

To aid the recovery, in its final phase, TDD employs behavioral activation (Jacobson, Martell, and Dimidjian 2001) in order to activate motivation through the experience of pleasure and to increase self-efficacy by engaging the patient in pleasurable activities. Altogether, TDD comprises three phases: exploration, acceptance, and behavioral activation. In its initial two phases, it identifies and targets FLED (failure: loss, entrapment, defeat), the core drivers of depression, in order to help the transition from protest to acceptance. Identification of FLED is usually achieved through psychodynamic exploration, and acceptance – by practice of mindfulness; behavioral activation follows afterwards (Krupnik 2014). More recently, TDD has been integrated with Eye Movement Desensitization and Reprocessing (EMDR), another experiential therapy (Shapiro 2017), to form TDD-EMDR therapy for depression (Krupnik 2015b, a, 2018a). In TDD-EMDR, EMDR intervention substitutes mindfulness in the acceptance phase while leaving the overall structure and strategy of TDD unchanged.

4.2. Predictive Coding as a Target for Therapy in Depression

In Predictive Processing Framework (PPF), malfunction of predictive coding or false inference is considered the source of psychopathology (Friston et al. 2014). Various therapies for depression have been conceptualized within this paradigm. The anti-depressant effects of serotonin and dopamine enhancing medications have been related to restoration of the accurate generative models of reward (Chekroud 2015). The former was hypothesized to restore reward-sensitivity through increasing reward-related prediction error's precision; the latter – to restore the optimal rate of reward learning through increasing synaptic efficacy. In the same article, Chekroud suggests that the mechanism of behavioral activation and interpersonal therapies is modification of active inference. Helping depressed people change their negatively biased sampling of the environment into a more positive one is expected to correct their negatively biased generative model of the world through learning more accurate, empirical priors.

At the level of interoception, deep brain stimulation of anterior cingulate cortex has been hypothesized to exert its anti-depressant through its top-down effect on allostatic priors, whereas vagal nerve stimulation is thought to help depression by increasing the precision of interoceptive prediction errors (Barrett, Quigley, and Hamilton 2016). Of special relevance to iESP model is suggestion by Stephan, et al. (Stephan et al. 2016) that physical activity may be therapeutic (for fatigue) because it increases self-efficacy. A recent overview of psychotherapy in PPF terms has recently been offered (Holmes and Nolte 2019).

How can we understand TDD therapy in PPF? Its first, exploratory phase examines the patient's depressive generative model of himself in the inimical world. The objective is to identify the most affectively salient FLED, because it is the likeliest driver of protest and, consequently, interoceptive allostatic predictions. In the above example of bereavement, such protest would be denial of irreversibility of the loss. Once identified, the patient is helped to accept the FLED in the following acceptance phase. Successful acceptance means a high precision of the *self-inefficacy* prior, hence the end of protest or, in clinical sense, *true* hopelessness. At this point, interoceptive allostasis priors are also at their highest precision, and the DSR has reached its lowest point. The acceptance step is supposed to meet two objectives. One is related to ceasing the protest, whose end will also terminate the allostatic pressure on interoceptive priors (Figure 1, 3). The other is to generate a predictive error contradicting the self-inefficacy prior; an act of acceptance (as any self-generated action, mental or physical) fosters a sense of agency and with it *self-efficacy* – once accepted, failure is no longer final.

The combination of cessation of protest and of the nascent increase in self-efficacy may create an opening for a greater sensitivity to prediction error by both the self-inefficacy meta-prior and interoceptive allostasis priors (Figure 3). This opening is then exploited in the third, behavioral activation, phase of TDD. The patient is encouraged to schedule and implement activities that can generate more and more prediction error, i.e., activities fulfilling self-efficacy (fostering the feelings of competency and accomplishment) and disconfirming the stress priors (pleasurable, relaxing, stimulating). In the absence of allostatic pressure, the precision of stress and self-inefficacy priors is likely to relax further, which would lead to increased precision of prediction errors, in which case the depressive generative model along with DSR will invert (Figure 3).

From the above description, acceptance emerges as a crucial step in TDD therapy. It is achieved either through practice of mindfulness in TDD (Krupnik 2014) or using EMDR interventions in TDD-EMDR (Krupnik

2015b, a, 2018a). In both cases, acceptance is understood as 'giving up' on protest through accepting the irreversible nature of FLED. It is worth repeating here the Clark and colleagues conclusion that, "...major depression occurs when the brain is certain that it will encounter an uncertain environment, i.e., the world is inherently volatile, capricious, unpredictable and uncontrollable." (Clark, Watson, and Friston 2018), p 2278). In this sense, acceptance introduces a degree of certainty (irreversibility of failure) into the mental representation of unpredictable world. Notably, in TDD-EMDR, decrease of depressive symptoms correlates with increase in the accepting attitude (Figure 4, Krupnik 2018a).

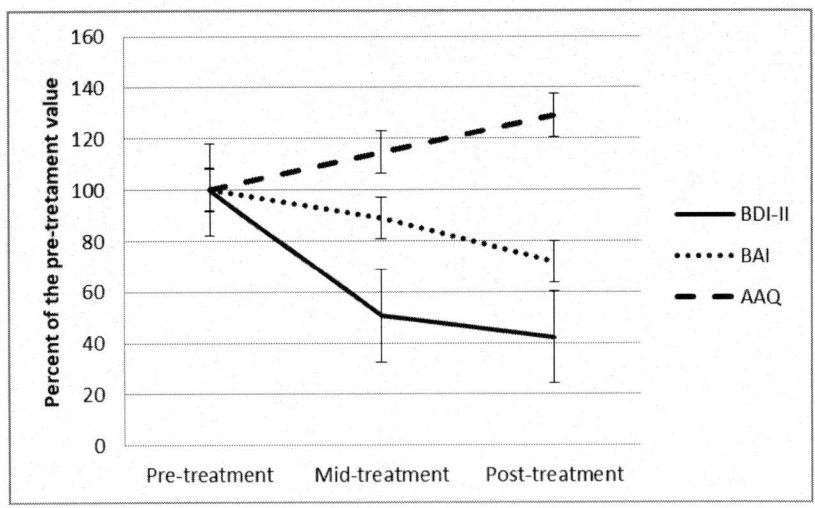

Figure 4. The dynamics of patient's scores in the course of TDD-EMDR therapy. AAQ – Acceptance and Action Questionnaire, BDI-II – Beck's Depression Inventory, BAI – Beck's Anxiety Inventory. Error bars show Standard Errors.

4.3. Strategic Modification of Priors (SMOP) as a Universal Integrative Therapy

The conception of psychopathology as false inference (Friston et al. 2014) implies that the mechanism of change in therapy is learning a new, more accurate, inference. Therefore, the objective of therapeutic intervention is to help the patient's generative model correct its biased predictions. In Bayesian terms, it means return to the optimal inference about the world and self given the available statistics. In order to successfully negotiate environmental challenges minimization of uncertainty should go along with optimizing adaptation. Optimal adaptation can be understood as an efficient energy metabolism sustaining minimal entropy. The combination of minimal informational entropy (uncertainty) with minimal structural entropy could be an operational definition of health, including mental health. This idea has been intuitively known since antiquity as expressed by the Roman poet Juvenal, "a healthy mind in a healthy body" (356 AD). In iEPS model of depression, this would mean helping depressive generative model learn optimal precision weighting and active inference.

Although a number of therapeutic interventions (including psycho-, pharmaco-, and electrophysiological therapy) have been framed in PPF terms, as reviewed in the previous section, only in one instance, to my knowledge, has PPF been explicitly used as a theoretical basis for therapy development (Krupnik and Cherkasova 2018). In that work, a behavioral intervention was specifically designed to generate a prediction error targeting the presumed pathogenic prior in a case of motor movement conversion disorder. That stategy was dubbed Strategic Modification of Priors (SMOP).

Later, SMOP was integrated with nested hierarchy principle for psychotherapy integration (Krupnik 2019a). The main premises of the principle are that all therapies are integrative, since 'mono-therapy' is more an abstraction than reality; that integrative therapy is co-constructed in a therapeutic encounter, and that, therefore, regarding therapies as intervention sets rather than manualized brands may be a more accurate representation of real-life therapy (Krupnik 2018b). Accordingly, the author suggests heuristic rules for assembling an integrative therapy, where it is structured following a top down hierarchy (Figure 5). On top of it is the strategic decision about the master goal: change vs maintenance. One step down is a theory of pathology in a given case, further down is a theory of a presumed mechanism of change that is informed by the theory of pathology, and at the bottom is a choice of intervention informed by the theory of the mechanism of change (Krupnik 2018b).

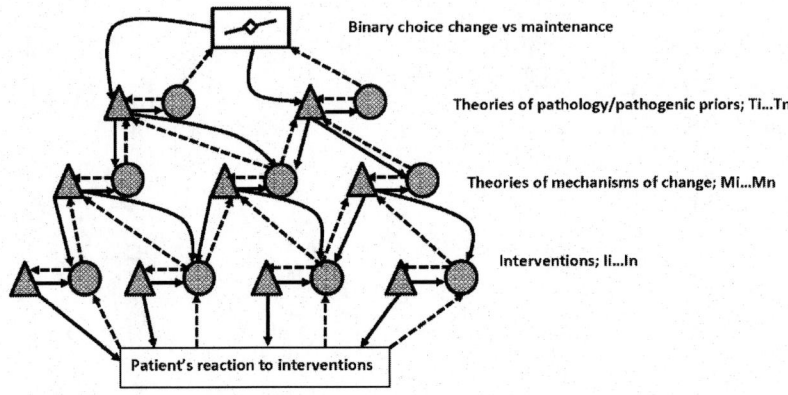

Figure 5. Predictive processing model of the hierarchical nest of universal (SMOP) psychotherapy (modified from Krupnik, 2017, 2019a). (Also, compare to Figure 2).

Therapy is co-created during a therapeutic encounter, where the therapist's generative model of the encounter generates predictions (theories) about the patient's needs and pathogenic priors, and about interventions' mechanisms and efficacy. Patient's reactions to the interventions provide a bottom-up stream of feedback that either confirms and reinforces the predictions or generates prediction error. The latter is then suppressed by the therapist through adjusting his theories and interventions. Importantly, everything a therapist does in session (specific techniques and social transactions, consciously or unconsciously) is considered intervention. (Patient's generative model is not shown here.)
▲ Prediction unit, ● Error unit, ⎯⎯ Top-down prediction signaling, ⎯ ⎯ Bottom-up error signaling.

In SMOP, theoretical case conceptualization includes identification of aberrant extero- and interoceptive predictions and imbalance in precision weighting. Their adjustment constitutes the mechanism of change, and interventions are chosen to facilitate it (Krupnik 2019a). Importantly, the hierarchical nest of integrative therapy itself functions as a Bayesian generative model (Figure 5). The model generates predictions about the causes of the observed symptoms; it also predicts how they may change in response to intervention. The patient's response then generates prediction error to either confirm or disconfirm the predictions, and the model of therapeutic encounter adjusts accordingly (Krupnik 2019a). Of note, real-life therapy, as any social encounter, is an evolving process of interaction between the therapist's and patient's generative models.

Next, I want to offer an interpretation of TDD hierarchical nest from the SMOP perspective. In the exploratory phase, TDD develops a theory of the patient's failure, identifying the exteroceptive priors driving his protest and the dynamics of his self-efficacy meta-prior. Then, it targets them with acceptance-fostering interventions through either mindfulness, as in TDD, or EMDR, as in TDD-EMDR, expecting the protest to stop. The following behavioral activation phase is expected to generate interoceptive prediction error targeting the stress priors.

Mindfulness intervention appears rather intuitive: mindful observance of one's failure presumes a low reactivity, affective distancing, and distributed attention, all of which can lead to decrease of exteroceptive PE precision weighting. This may help increase the precision of self-efficacy meta-prior, as discussed in the previous section.

The role of EMDR intervention, on the other hand, is less obvious. Despite multiple theories about the mechanism of action of EMDR's core intervention, saccadic eye movements (or other kinds of bi-lateral stimulation (BLS), there is no clear understanding of how they work (for a recent review see Landin-Romero et al. 2018). I suggest that PPF offers a straightforward and most parsimonious hypothesis about therapeutic action of BLS. In EMDR, patients are asked to focus on affectively charged negative memories/thoughts/images while BLS is applied (Shapiro 2017). It is possible that juxtaposition of negative imagery with unrelated sensory stimulation generates a prediction error that is propagated up the information processing hierarchy (Figure 2), affecting the network of prior beliefs constituting the negative memory. A similar theory of BLS action has recently been formulated (Chamberlin 2019). Consistent with this hypothesis, there are reports on therapeutic effects of other than BLS sensory-motor stimulation (Krupnik and Cherkasova 2018, Holmes et al. 2009). The key to sensory-motor interventions appears to be in pairing exposure to negative material with incongruent stimulation creating prediction error.

CONCLUSION

This chapter describes an emerging integrative model of psychopathology of depression, iESP (Figure 3), which considers depression an arrested depressive response to stress or DSR. I suggest that the model is applicable to all disorders of stress response, which would include a majority of psychiatric conditions. One of the advantages of iESP is that it is a *clinical-level* theory, since it links the hypothesized mechanisms of pathology to their clinical manifestations. The importance of having a clinical-level theory is its direct applicability to practice as reviewed in the sections describing therapies for depression.

Historically, all psychotherapy is theory-based, which can be traced in its brand names, e.g., psychoanalysis is based on psychoanalytical theory, cognitive and behavioral therapy on cognitive and behavioral theories, respectively, etc. Therapies that initially sprang from serendipitous discoveries have, too, developed a theory to back them up, e.g., adaptive information processing theory for EMDR (Shapiro 2017) or intention-attention-attitude theory for Mindfulness-Based Stress Reduction (Shapiro et al. 2006). It has also been noted that more recent innovations in psychotherapy are more technique than theory-driven, which may impede its progress (Schweiger et al. 2019).

Lately, much emphasis has shifted toward the question of therapy efficacy. Randomized controlled trials have become a rite of passage for therapies into the distinguished league of *evidence-based* practices with Cochrane Database of Systematic Reviews as the gate keeper. Yet, when different therapies, especially evidence-supported ones, are compared they tend to be of similar efficacy, a phenomenon known as Dodo Bird verdict, which is believed to be due to a relatively large effect of *common factors* that are not specific to therapeutic techniques (Wampold 2015). This raises a possibility that further innovation in psychotherapeutic techniques may have a diminished return relative to the resources spent. Consistent with this idea is the finding that in the last three decades psychotherapies for depression have not become any more efficacious (Cuijpers et al. 2019).

I suggested before that there were as many therapies as there were therapeutic encounters (Krupnik 2018b). This idea is not new and has been advanced as contextual model of therapy (Wampold 2001). This brings up a possibility that further progress in psychotherapy may lie not as much in theoretical or technical innovations but in increasing treatment specificity. This premise has been aptly captured long ago in Gordon Paul's (Paul 1967) cornerstone question: "what treatment, by whom, is most effective for this individual with that specific problem, and under which set of circumstances?" Currently, this concept is known as precision medicine.

What methodology can be used to increase the specificity of psychosocial treatments? One recently advocated option is heuristically-driven psychotherapy as described in the Bayesian model of integrative psychotherapy or SMOP (Krupnik 2018b, 2019a). In that model, therapist is not a delivery vehicle for a manualized treatment but a generative model of the treatment, generating predictions and resolving prediction errors through active therapeutic inference and learning (Figure 5). The ability to flexibly optimize such predictive processing in order to co-create with the patient a highly specific and effective therapy can be an operational definition of therapeutic mastery.

REFERENCES

American Psychiatric Association. (2013). *Diagnostic and statistical manual of mental disorders* (5th ed.). Arlington, VA: American Psychiatric Publishing.

Andrews, Paul W., and Zachary Durisko. 2017. "The evolution of depressive phenotypes." In *The Oxford handbook of mood disorders*, edited by DeRubeis & Strunk, 24-36. New York, NY: Oxford University Press.

Ashby, W. R., 1947. "Principles of the self-organizing dynamic system." *Journal of General Psychology* 37:125-128.

Badcock, Paul B., Christopher G. Davey, Sarah Whittle, Nicholas B. Allen, and Karl J. Friston. 2017. "The Depressed Brain: An Evolutionary Systems Theory." *Trends in Cognitive Sciences* 21 (3):182-194. doi: https://doi.org/10.1016/j.tics.2017.01.005.

Bandura, Albert. 1977. "Self-efficacy: Toward a unifying theory of behavioral change." *Psychological Review* 84 (2):191-215. doi: 10.1037/0033-295X.84.2.191.

Barrett, Lisa Feldman, Karen S. Quigley, and Paul Hamilton. 2016. "An active inference theory of allostasis and interoception in depression." *Phil. Trans. R. Soc. B* 371 (1708):1-17. doi: 10.1098/rstb.2016.0011.

Barton, Scott. 1994. "Chaos, self-organization, and psychology." *American Psychologist* 49 (1):5-14.

Beck, A. T. 1967. *Depression: clinical, experimental, and theoretical aspects*. New York: Hoeber Medical Division, Harper & Row.

Berzoff, J., and M. Hayes. 1996. "Biopsychosocial Aspects of Depression." In *Inside out and outside in: psychodynamic clinical theory and practice in contemporary multicultural contexts*, edited by J. Berzoff, L. M. Flanagan and P. Hertz, 365-396. Northvale, NJ: Jason Aronson, Inc.

Blatt, Sidney J., Joseph P. D'Afflitti, and Donald M. Quinlan. 1976. "Experiences of depression in normal young adults." *Journal of Abnormal Psychology* 85 (4):383-389. doi: 10.1037/0021-843X.85.4.383.

Bleuler, Manfred. 1963. "Conception of schizophrenia within the last fifty years and today [abridged]."

Bogdan, R., Y. S. Nikolova, and D. A. Pizzagalli. 2012. "Neurogenetics of depression: a focus on reward processing and stress sensitivity." *Neurobiol Dis* 52:12-23.

Boonstra, Nynke, Rianne Klaassen, Sjoerd Sytema, Max Marshall, Lieuwe De Haan, Lex Wunderink, and Durk Wiersma. 2012. "Duration of untreated psychosis and negative symptoms—a systematic review and meta-analysis of individual patient data." *Schizophrenia research* 142 (1-3):12-19. doi: https://doi.org/10.1016/j.schres.2012.08.017.

Bowlby, J. 1980. *Loss: Sadness and Depression*. 3 vols. Vol. 3, *Attachment and Loss*. New York: Basic Books.

Brown, Charlotte, Herbert C. Schulberg, Michael J. Madonia, M. Katherine Shear, and Patricia R. Houck. 1996. "Treatment outcomes for primary care patients with major depression and lifetime anxiety disorders." *The American Journal of Psychiatry* 153 (10):1293-1300. doi: 10.1176/ajp.153.10.1293.

Cannon, Walter B. 1929. "Organization for physiological homeostasis." *Physiological reviews* 9 (3):399-431. doi: https://doi.org/10.1152/physrev.1929.9.3.399.

Chamberlin, D. Eric. 2019. "The Predictive Processing Model of EMDR." *Frontiers in Psychology* 10 (2267). doi: 10.3389/fpsyg.2019.02267.

Chang, W. C., Christy L. M. Hui, Jennifer Y. M. Tang, Gloria H. Y. Wong, May M. L. Lam, Sherry K. W. Chan, and Eric Y. H. Chen. 2011. "Persistent negative symptoms in first-episode schizophrenia: a prospective three-year follow-up study." *Schizophrenia research* 133 (1-3):22-28. doi: https://doi.org/10.1016/j.schres.2011.09.006.

Chekroud, Adam M. 2015. "Unifying treatments for depression: an application of the Free Energy Principle." *Frontiers in Psychology* 6 (153). doi: 10.3389/fpsyg.2015.00153.

Clark, Andy. 2013. "Whatever next? Predictive brains, situated agents, and the future of cognitive science." *Behavioral and brain sciences* 36 (3):181-204. doi: doi:10.1017/S0140525X12000477.

Clark, James E., Stuart Watson, and Karl J. Friston. 2018. "What is mood? A computational perspective." *Psychological Medicine* 48 (14):2277-2284. doi: 10.1017/S0033291718000430.

Clayton, Paula J., William M. Grove, William Coryell, Martin Keller, Robert Hirschfeld, and Jan Fawcett. 1991. "Follow-up and family study of anxious depression." *Am J Psychiatry* 148 (11):1512-1517.

Cryan, John F., Cedric Mombereau, and Annick Vassout. 2005. "The tail suspension test as a model for assessing antidepressant activity: review of pharmacological and genetic studies in mice." *Neuroscience &*

Biobehavioral Reviews 29 (4-5):571-625. doi: https://doi.org/10.1016/j.neubiorev.2005.03.009.

Cuijpers, P., E. Karyotaki, M. Reijnders, and D. D. Ebert. 2019. "Was Eysenck right after all? A reassessment of the effects of psychotherapy for adult depression." *Epidemiology and psychiatric sciences* 28 (1):21-30. doi: https://doi.org/10.1017/S2045796018000057.

Dennison, Meg J., Maya L. Rosen, Kelly A. Sambrook, Jessica L. Jenness, Margaret A. Sheridan, and Katie A. McLaughlin. 2019. "Differential Associations of Distinct Forms of Childhood Adversity With Neurobehavioral Measures of Reward Processing: A Developmental Pathway to Depression." *Child Development* 90 (1):e96-e113. doi: 10.1111/cdev.13011.

Dimidjian, S., S. D. Hollon, K. S. Dobson, K. B. Schmaling, R. J. Kohlenberg, M. E. Addis, R. Gallop, J. B. McGlinchey, D. K. Markley, J. K. Gollan, D. C. Atkins, D. L. Dunner, and N. S. Jacobson. 2006. "Randomized trial of behavioral activation, cognitive therapy, and antidepressant medication in the acute treatment of adults with major depression." *J Consult Clin Psychol* 74 (4):658-70. doi: http://dx.doi.org/10.1037/0022-006X.74.4.658.

Disner, Seth G., Christopher G. Beevers, Emily A. P. Haigh, and Aaron T. Beck. 2011. "Neural mechanisms of the cognitive model of depression." *Nature Reviews Neuroscience* 12 (8):467-477. doi: 10.1038/nrn3027.

Dołęga, Krzysztof. 2018. "Commentary: M-Autonomy." *Frontiers in psychology* 9:680-680. doi: 10.3389/fpsyg.2018.00680.

Edwards, Mark J., Rick A. Adams, Harriet Brown, Isabel Pareés, and Karl J. Friston. 2012. "A Bayesian account of 'hysteria'." *Brain* 135 (11):3495-3512. doi: 10.1093/brain/aws129.

Fava, M. 2003. "Diagnosis and definition of treatment-resistant depression." *Biological Psychiatry* 53 (8):649-59.

Feldman, Harriet, and Karl Friston. 2010. "Attention, Uncertainty, and Free-Energy." *Frontiers in Human Neuroscience* 4 (215). doi: 10.3389/fnhum.2010.00215.

Ferrari, Alize J., Fiona J. Charlson, Rosana E. Norman, Scott B. Patten, Greg Freedman, Christopher J. L. Murray, Theo Vos, and Harvey A Whiteford. 2013. "Burden of depressive disorders by country, sex, age, and year: findings from the global burden of disease study 2010." *PLoS medicine* 10 (11):e1001547. doi: 10.1371/journal.pmed.1001547.

Ferrari, F., and R. F. Villa. 2017. "The Neurobiology of Depression: an Integrated Overview from Biological Theories to Clinical Evidence." *Molecular Neurobiology* 54 (7):4847-4865. doi: 10.1007/s12035-016-0032-y.

Freud, Sigmund. 1966. *The complete introductory lectures on psychoanalysis*. Translated by James Strachey. New York: W. W. Norton & Company, Inc.

Friston, Karl. 2010. "The free-energy principle: a unified brain theory?" *Nat Rev Neurosci* 11 (2):127-138. doi: 10.1038/nrn2787.

Friston, Karl J, Klaas Enno Stephan, Read Montague, and Raymond J Dolan. 2014. "Computational psychiatry: the brain as a phantastic organ." *The Lancet Psychiatry* 1 (2):148-158. doi: https://doi.org/10.1016/S2215-0366(14)70275-5.

Friston, Karl J., Tamara Shiner, Thomas FitzGerald, Joseph M. Galea, Rick Adams, Harriet Brown, Raymond J. Dolan, Rosalyn Moran, Klaas Enno Stephan, and Sven Bestmann. 2012. "Dopamine, Affordance and Active Inference." *PLOS Computational Biology* 8 (1):e1002327. doi: 10.1371/journal.pcbi.1002327.

Friston, Karl, James Kilner, and Lee Harrison. 2006. "A free energy principle for the brain." *Journal of Physiology-Paris* 100 (1):70-87. doi: https://doi.org/10.1016/j.jphysparis.2006.10.001.

Furukawa, T. A., T. Kitamura, and K. Takahashi. 2000. "Time to recovery of an inception cohort with hitherto untreated unipolar major depressive episodes." *British Journal Psychiatry* 177:331-5.

Gilbert, Paul. 2000. "The relationship of shame, social anxiety and depression: The role of the evaluation of social rank." *Clinical Psychology & Psychotherapy* 7 (3):174-189.

Giosan, Cezar, Oana Cobeanu, Cristina Mogoase, Vlad Muresan, Loretta S Malta, Katarzyna Wyka, and Aurora Szentagotai. 2014. "Evolutionary cognitive therapy versus standard cognitive therapy for depression: a protocol for a blinded, randomized, superiority clinical trial." *Trials* 15 (1):83. doi: doi:10.1186/1745-6215-15-83.

Gold, Mark S., A. L. C. Pottash, and I. R. L. Extein. 1981. "Hypothyroidism and depression: evidence from complete thyroid function evaluation." *Jama* 245 (19):1919-1922. doi: 10.1001/jama.1981.03310440019016.

Grimby, A. 1993. "Bereavement among elderly people: grief reactions, post-bereavement hallucinations and quality of life." *Acta Psychiatrica Scandinavica* 87 (1):72-80. doi: 10.1111/j.1600-0447.1993.tb03332.x.

Hagen, E. H. 1999. "The Functions of Postpartum Depression." *Evolution and Human Behavior* 20 (5):325–359. doi: https://doi.org/10.1016/S1090-5138(99)00016-1.

Hayes, S. C., K. Strosahl, and K. G. Wilson. 1999. *Acceptance and commitment therapy: An experiential approach to behavior change*. New York: Guilford Press.

Holmes, Emily A., Ella L. James, Thomas Coode-Bate, and Catherine Deeprose. 2009. "Can Playing the Computer Game "Tetris" Reduce the Build-Up of Flashbacks for Trauma? A Proposal from Cognitive Science." *PLOS ONE* 4 (1):e4153. doi: 10.1371/journal.pone.0004153.

Holmes, Jeremy, and Tobias Nolte. 2019. ""Surprise" and the Bayesian Brain: Implications for Psychotherapy Theory and Practice." *Frontiers in Psychology* 10 (592). doi: 10.3389/fpsyg.2019.00592.

Hosoya, Toshihiko, Stephen A. Baccus, and Markus Meister. 2005. "Dynamic predictive coding by the retina." *Nature* 436 (7047):71-77. doi: 10.1038/nature03689.

Huang, Yanping, and Rajesh P. N. Rao. 2011. "Predictive coding." *Wiley Interdisciplinary Reviews: Cognitive Science* 2 (5):580-593. doi: 10.1002/wcs.142.

Jacobson, N. S., C. R. Martell, and S. Dimidjian. 2001. "Behavioral activation treatment for depression: Returning to contextual roots." *Clin Psychol Sci Prac* 8:255-270.

Joffily, Mateus, and Giorgio Coricelli. 2013. "Emotional Valence and the Free-Energy Principle." *PLOS Computational Biology* 9 (6):e100 3094. doi: 10.1371/journal.pcbi.1003094.

Jorm, AF, NB Allen, AJ Morgan, and R Purcell. 2009. *A Guide to What Works for Depression*. Melbourne: beyondblue.

Karsten, Julie, Catharina A. Hartman, Johannes H. Smit, Frans G. Zitman, Aartjan T. F. Beekman, Pim Cuijpers, A. J. Willem van der Does, Johan Ormel, Willem A. Nolen, and Brenda W. J. H. Penninx. 2018. "Psychiatric history and subthreshold symptoms as predictors of the occurrence of depressive or anxiety disorder within 2 years." *British Journal of Psychiatry* 198 (3):206-212. doi: 10.1192/bjp.bp. 110.080572.

Katz, Richard J. 1982. "Animal model of depression: Pharmacological sensitivity of a hedonic deficit." *Pharmacology Biochemistry and Behavior* 16 (6):965-968. doi: https://doi.org/10.1016/0091-3057(82)90053-3.

Kaufman, I. Ch., and L. A. Rosenblum. 1967. "The reaction to separation in infant monkeys: Anaclitic depression and conservation-Withdrawal." *Psychosomatic Medicine* 29 (6):648-75.

Keller, M. B., P. W. Lavori, T. I. Mueller, J. Endicott, W. Coryell, R. M. Hirschfeld, and T. Shea. 1992. "Time to recovery, chronicity, and levels of psychopathology in major depression. A 5-year prospective follow-up of 431 subjects." *Archives of General Psychiatry* 49 (10):809-16.

Kessler, R. C., P. Berglund, O. Demler, R. Jin, K. R. Merikangas, and E. E. Walters. 2005. "Lifetime prevalence and age-of-onset distributions of DSM-IV disorders in the National Comorbidity Survey Replication." *Archives of General Psychiatry* 62 (6):593-602.

Kessler, R. C., C. B. Nelson, K. A. McGonagle, and J. Liu. 1996. "Comorbidity of DSM-III-R major depressive disorder in the general population: Results from the US National Comorbidity Survey." *British Journal of Psychiatry* 168 (30):17-30.

Kessler, Ronald C., and William J. Magee. 2009. "Childhood adversities and adult depression: basic patterns of association in a US national survey." *Psychological Medicine* 23 (3):679-690. doi: 10.1017/S0033291700025460.

Khalid, Arshi, Byung Sun Kim, Bo Am Seo, Soon-Tae Lee, Keun-Hwa Jung, Kon Chu, Sang Kun Lee, and Daejong Jeon. 2016. "Gamma oscillation in functional brain networks is involved in the spontaneous remission of depressive behavior induced by chronic restraint stress in mice." *BMC Neuroscience* 17 (1):4. doi: 10.1186/s12868-016-0239-x.

Klerman, GL, MM Weissman, BJ Rounsaville, and ES Chevron. 1984. *Interpersonal psychotherapy of depression, Northvale, NJ: Jason Aronson.*

Koolhaas, J. M., P. M. Hermann, C. Kemperman, B. Bohus, R. H. v. d. Hoofdakker, and D. G. M. Beersma. 1990. "Single social interaction leading to defeat in male rats induces a gradual, but long lasting behavioral change: a model of depression?" *Neuroscience Research Communication* 7:35-41.

Krupnik, Valery. 2014. "A Novel Therapeutic Frame for Treating Depression in Group Treating Depression Downhill." *SAGE Open* 4 (1):1-12. doi: 10.1177/2158244014523793.

Krupnik, Valery. 2015a. "Integrating EMDR Into a Novel Evolutionary-Based Therapy for Depression: A Case Study of Postpartum Depression." *Journal of EMDR Practice and Research* 9 (3):137-149.

Krupnik, Valery. 2015b. "Integrating EMDR into an evolutionary-based therapy for depression: a case study." *Clinical case reports* 3 (5):301-307. doi: 10.1002/ccr3.228.

Krupnik, Valery. 2018a. "Differential Effects of an Evolutionary-Based EMDR Therapy on Depression and Anxiety Symptoms: A Case Series Study." *Journal of EMDR Practice and Research* 12 (2):46-57. doi: 10. 1891/ 1933- 3196. 12. 2. 46.

Krupnik, Valery. 2018b. "Nested Hierarchy for Therapy Integration: Integrating the Integrative." *International Journal of Integrative Psychotherapy* 8:40-78.

Krupnik, Valery. 2018c. "Trauma or adversity?" *Traumatology*. doi: http://dx.doi.org/10.1037/trm0000169.

Krupnik, Valery. 2019a. "Bayesian Approach to Psychotherapy Integration: Strategic Modification of Priors." *Frontiers in Psychology* 10 (356). doi: 10.3389/fpsyg.2019.00356.

Krupnik, Valery. 2019b. "A Different EMDR: Treating Depressive disorders with TDD-EMDR." EMDRIA 2019, Garden Grove, CA.

Krupnik, Valery, and Mariya V Cherkasova. 2018. "Strategic Symptom Displacement in Therapy of a Motor Conversion Disorder Comorbid with PTSD: Case Presentation." *Journal of Contemporary Psychotherapy*: 1-8. doi: https://doi.org/10.1007/s10879-018-9408-9.

Kübler-Ross, Elisabeth. 1997. *On death and dying*. New York: Simon and Schuster.

Landin-Romero, Ramon, Ana Moreno-Alcazar, Marco Pagani, and Benedikt L. Amann. 2018. "How Does Eye Movement Desensitization and Reprocessing Therapy Work? A Systematic Review on Suggested Mechanisms of Action." *Frontiers in Psychology* 9 (1395). doi: 10.3389/fpsyg.2018.01395.

Lawson, Rebecca P., Geraint Rees, and Karl J. Friston. 2014. "An aberrant precision account of autism." *Frontiers in Human Neuroscience* 8 (302). doi: 10.3389/fnhum.2014.00302.

McEwen, Bruce S, and John C Wingfield. 2003. "The concept of allostasis in biology and biomedicine." *Hormones and behavior* 43 (1):2-15. doi: https://doi.org/10.1016/S0018-506X(02)00024-7.

McGonagle, Katherine A., and Ronald C. Kessler. 1990. "Chronic stress, acute stress, and depressive symptoms." *American Journal of Community Psychology* 18 (5):681-706. doi: 10.1007/bf00931237.

McIntosh, Andrew M., Patrick F. Sullivan, and Cathryn M. Lewis. 2019. "Uncovering the Genetic Architecture of Major Depression." *Neuron* 102 (1):91-103. doi: https://doi.org/10.1016/j.neuron.2019.03.022.

Mobus, George E, and Michael C Kalton. 2015. *Principles of systems science*. New York, NY: Springer.

Monroe, Scott M, and Kate L Harkness. 2005. "Life stress, the" kindling" hypothesis, and the recurrence of depression: considerations from a life stress perspective." *Psychological review* 112 (2):417-445.

Moskowitz, Andrew K. 2004. "Scared Stiff": Catatonia as an Evolutionary-Based Fear Response." *Psychological Review* 111 (4):984-1002. doi: 10.1037/0033-295X.111.4.984.

Moutoussis, Michael, Pasco Fearon, Wael El-Deredy, Raymond J. Dolan, and Karl J. Friston. 2014. "Bayesian inferences about the self (and others): A review." *Consciousness and Cognition* 25 (Supplement C):67-76. doi: https://doi.org/10.1016/j.concog.2014.01.009.

Mullur, Rashmi, Yan-Yun Liu, and Gregory A Brent. 2014. "Thyroid hormone regulation of metabolism." *Physiological reviews* 94 (2):355-382. doi: https://doi.org/10.1152/physrev.00030.2013.

Nesse, R. M. 2000. "Is depression an adaptation?" *Archives of General Psychiatry* 57 (1):14-20.

Nestler, E. J., and W. A. Carlezon, Jr. 2006. "The mesolimbic dopamine reward circuit in depression." *Biological Psychiatry* 59 (12):1151-9.

Northoff, Georg, Christine Wiebking, Todd Feinberg, and Jaak Panksepp. 2011. "The 'resting-state hypothesis' of major depressive disorder—A translational subcortical–cortical framework for a system disorder." *Neuroscience & Biobehavioral Reviews* 35 (9):1929-1945. doi: https://doi.org/10.1016/j.neubiorev.2010.12.007.

Oken, Barry S., Irina Chamine, and Wayne Wakeland. 2015. "A systems approach to stress, stressors and resilience in humans." *Behavioural brain research* 282:144-154. doi: https://doi.org/10.1016/j.bbr.2014.12.047.

Parker, G. 2007. "Is depression overdiagnosed? Yes." *British Medical Journal* 335 (7615):328.

Parker, G., K. Roy, and K. Eyers. 2003. "Cognitive behavior therapy for depression? Choose horses for courses." *Am J Psychiatry* 160 (5):825-34.

Paul, G. L. 1967. "Strategy of outcome research in psychotherapy." *Journal of Consulting Psychology* 31 (2):109-118. doi: 10.1037/h0024436.

Paulus, Martin P., and Murray B. Stein. 2010. "Interoception in anxiety and depression." *Brain Structure and Function* 214 (5):451-463. doi: 10.1007/s00429-010-0258-9.

Peters, Achim, Bruce S. McEwen, and Karl Friston. 2017. "Uncertainty and stress: Why it causes diseases and how it is mastered by the brain." *Progress in Neurobiology* 156:164-188. doi: https://doi.org/10.1016/j.pneurobio.2017.05.004.

Pollatos, Olga, Eva Traut-Mattausch, and Rainer Schandry. 2009. "Differential effects of anxiety and depression on interoceptive accuracy." *Depression and Anxiety* 26 (2):167-173. doi: 10.1002/da.20504.

Powers, A. R., C. Mathys, and P. R. Corlett. 2017. "Pavlovian conditioning–induced hallucinations result from overweighting of perceptual priors." *Science* 357 (6351):596-600. doi: 10.1126/science.aan3458.

Price, J., L. Sloman, R. Gardner, Jr., P. Gilbert, and P. Rohde. 1994. "The social competition hypothesis of depression." *British Journal of Psychiatry* 164 (3):309-15.

Rai, D., P. Zitko, K. Jones, J. Lynch, and R. Araya. 2013. "Country- and individual-level socioeconomic determinants of depression: multilevel cross-national comparison." *Br J Psychiatry* 202 (3):195-203.

Rao, Rajesh P. N., and Dana H. Ballard. 1999. "Predictive coding in the visual cortex: a functional interpretation of some extra-classical receptive-field effects." *Nature Neuroscience* 2 (1):79-87. doi: 10.1038/4580.

Ray, Partho Sarothi, Jie Jia, Peng Yao, Mithu Majumder, Maria Hatzoglou, and Paul L. Fox. 2009. "A stress-responsive RNA switch regulates VEGFA expression." *Nature* 457 (7231):915-919. doi: 10.1038/nature07598.

Robins, Clive J, and Paul Block. 1989. "Cognitive theories of depression viewed from a diathesis-stress perspective: Evaluations of the models of Beck and of Abramson, Seligman, and Teasdale." *Cognitive Therapy and Research* 13 (4):297-313. doi: https://doi.org/10.1007/BF01173475.

Schweiger, Janina Isabel, Kai G. Kahl, Jan Philipp Klein, Valerija Sipos, and Ulrich Schweiger. 2019. "Innovation in Psychotherapy,

Challenges, and Opportunities: An Opinion Paper." *Frontiers in psychology* 10:495-495. doi: 10.3389/fpsyg.2019.00495.

Seligman, M. E. 1972. "Learned helplessness." *Annual Review of Medicine* 23:407-12.

Selye, Hans. 1956. *The stress of life*. New York: McCraw-Hill Book.

Seth, Anil K., and Karl J. Friston. 2016. "Active interoceptive inference and the emotional brain." *Philosophical Transactions of the Royal Society B: Biological Sciences* 371 (1708):20160007. doi: doi:10.1098/rstb.2016.0007.

Shapiro, F. 2017. *Eye Movement Desensitization and Reprocessing (EMDR) Therapy: Basic principles, protocols and procedures*. 3rd ed. New York: Guilford Press.

Shapiro, Shauna L., Linda E. Carlson, John A. Astin, and Benedict Freedman. 2006. "Mechanisms of mindfulness." *Journal of Clinical Psychology* 62 (3):373-386. doi: 10.1002/jclp.20237.

Shedler, J. 2010. "The efficacy of psychodynamic psychotherapy." *American Psychologist* 65 (2):98-109.

Solomon, David A., Martin B. Keller, Andrew C. Leon, Timothy I. Mueller, Philip W. Lavori, M. Shea, William Coryell, Meredith Warshaw, Carolyn Turvey, Jack D. Maser, and Jean Endicott. 2000. "Multiple recurrences of major depressive disorder." *The American Journal of Psychiatry* 157 (2):229-233.

Souery, D., and W. Pitchot. 2013. "Definitions and Predictors of Treatment-resistant Depression." In *Treatment-resistant Depression*, edited by S. Kasper and S. Montgomery, 1-20. John Wiley & Sons, Ltd.

Spijker, J., R. de Graaf, R. V. Bijl, A. T. Beekman, J. Ormel, and W. A. Nolen. 2002. "Duration of major depressive episodes in the general population: results from The Netherlands Mental Health Survey and Incidence Study (NEMESIS)." *British Journal of Psychiatry* 181:208-13.

Srinivasan, Mandyam Veerambudi, Simon Barry Laughlin, A. Dubs, and George Adrian Horridge. 1982. "Predictive coding: a fresh view of inhibition in the retina." *Proceedings of the Royal Society of London.*

Series B. Biological Sciences 216 (1205):427-459. doi: doi:10.1098/rspb.1982.0085.

Stephan, Klaas E., Zina M. Manjaly, Christoph D. Mathys, Lilian A. E. Weber, Saee Paliwal, Tim Gard, Marc Tittgemeyer, Stephen M. Fleming, Helene Haker, Anil K. Seth, and Frederike H. Petzschner. 2016. "Allostatic Self-efficacy: A Metacognitive Theory of Dyshomeostasis-Induced Fatigue and Depression." *Frontiers in Human Neuroscience* 10 (550). doi: 10.3389/fnhum.2016.00550.

Sterling, Peter. 2004. "Principles of Allostasis: Optimal Design, Predictive Regulation, Pathophysiology, and Rational Therapeutics." In *Allostasis, homeostasis, and the costs of physiological adaptation.*, edited by Jay Schulkin, 17-64. Cambridge University Press.

Strain, James J, and Michael Blumenfield. 2018. *Depression as a Systemic Illness*: Oxford University Press.

Syme, Kristen L., Zachary H. Garfield, and Edward H. Hagen. 2016. "Testing the bargaining vs. inclusive fitness models of suicidal behavior against the ethnographic record." *Evolution and Human Behavior* 37 (3):179-192. doi: https://doi.org/10.1016/j.evolhumbehav.2015.10.005.

Tang, Rong, Jian Wang, Lili Yang, Xiaohong Ding, Yufan Zhong, Jiexue Pan, Haiyan Yang, Liangshan Mu, Xia Chen, and Zimiao Chen. 2019. "Subclinical Hypothyroidism and Depression: A Systematic Review and Meta-Analysis." *Frontiers in endocrinology* 10:340-340. doi: 10.3389/fendo.2019.00340.

Tyedmers, Jens, Maria Lucia Madariaga, and Susan Lindquist. 2008. "Prion switching in response to environmental stress." *PLoS biology* 6 (11):e294. doi: https://doi.org/10.1371/journal.pbio.0060294.

Ursin, Holger, and Hege R Eriksen. 2004. "The cognitive activation theory of stress." *Psychoneuroendocrinology* 29 (5):567-592. doi: https://doi.org/10.1016/S0306-4530(03)00091-X.

Wakefield, J. C., and M. F. Schmitz. 2013. "When does depression become a disorder? Using recurrence rates to evaluate the validity of proposed changes in major depression diagnostic thresholds." *World Psychiatry* 12 (1):44-52.

Wampold, B. E. 2001. *The Great Psychotherapy Debate: Models, Methods, and Findings.* Mahwah, NJ: Lawrence Erlbaum.

Wampold, B. E. 2015. "How important are the common factors in psychotherapy? An update." *World Psychiatry* 14 (3):270-277. doi: 10.1002/wps.20238.

Watson, and P. W. Andrews. 2002. "Toward a revised evolutionary adaptationist analysis of depression: the social navigation hypothesis." *Journal of Affective Disorders* 72 (1):1-14.

Watt, D. F., and J. Panksepp. 2009. "Depression: An Evolutionarily Conserved Mechanism to Terminate Separation Distress? A Review of Aminergic, Peptidergic, and Neural Network Perspectives." *Neuropsychoanalysis* 11 (1):7-109.

Wilkinson, Sam, Guy Dodgson, and Kevin Meares. 2017. "Predictive Processing and the Varieties of Psychological Trauma." *Frontiers in Psychology* 8 (1840). doi: 10.3389/fpsyg.2017.01840.

Williams, J. M. G., J. D. Teasdale, Z. V. Segal, and J. Kabat-Zinn. 2007. *The mindful way through depression: Freeing yourself from chronic unhappiness.* New York: Guilford Press.

Wilsterman, Kathryn, C. Loren Buck, Brian M. Barnes, and Cory T. Williams. 2015. "Energy regulation in context: free-living female arctic ground squirrels modulate the relationship between thyroid hormones and activity among life history stages." *Hormones and behavior* 75:111-119. doi: https://doi.org/10.1016/j.yhbeh.2015.09.003.

Wolpert, L. 2008. "Depression in an evolutionary context." *Philosophy Ethics and Humanities in Medicine* 3:8.

Zellner, M. R., D. F. Watt, M. Solms, and J. Panksepp. 2011. "Affective neuroscientific and neuropsychoanalytic approaches to two intractable psychiatric problems: why depression feels so bad and what addicts really want." *Neuroscience and Biobehavioral Reviews* 35 (9):2000-8.

BIOGRAPHICAL SKETCH

Valery Krupnik, PhD

Affiliation: Department of Mental Health, Naval Hospital Camp Pendleton, Camp Pendleton, CA, US

Research and Professional Experience: psychotherapy practice and research; research in developmental biology and immunology.

Publications from the Last 3 Years:
Krupnik, V. (2019). Bayesian Approach to Psychotherapy Integration: Strategic Modification of Priors. *Frontiers in psychology*, *10*, 356.
Krupnik, V., & Cherkasova, M. V. (2018). Strategic Symptom Displacement in Therapy of a Motor Conversion Disorder Comorbid with PTSD: Case Presentation. *Journal of Contemporary Psychotherapy*, 1-8. https://doi.org/10.1007/s1087.
Krupnik, V. (2018). Trauma or adversity? *Traumatology*. http://dx.doi.org/10.1037/trm0000169.
Krupnik, V. (2018). Differential Effects of an Evolutionary-Based EMDR Therapy on Depression and Anxiety Symptoms: A Case Series Study. *Journal of EMDR Practice and Research*, *12*(2), 46-57.
Krupnik, V. (2018). Nested Hierarchy for Therapy Integration: Integrating the Integrative. *International Journal of Integrative Psychotherapy*, *8*, 40-78.

In: Depression and Anxiety
Editor: Shelley L. Becker

ISBN: 978-1-53617-229-4
© 2020 Nova Science Publishers, Inc.

Chapter 2

SEXUAL DYSFUNCTION AND DEPRESSION IN FEMALES

Swaleha Mujawar, Suprakash Chaudhury[*] *and Daniel Saldanha*
Department of Psychiatry, Dr. D. Y. Patil Medical College,
Dr. D. Y. Patil University, Pune, Maharshtra, India

ABSTRACT

A detailed search of the medical literature was conducted and articles from 1997-2009 were studied. Search methods included MEDLINE and PubMed databases for articles in English using search words of sexual dysfunction females/women, depression and depression and female sexual dysfunction. A total of 204 articles were screened for inclusion. Sexual problems and dissatisfaction with sex were commonly associated with depression. The prevalence of sexual problems in patients with depression is approximately twice that of the controls. Some of the antidepressants prescribed for depression may lead to impairment in the sexual functioning in all the phases of the sexual cycle. Antidepressant induced sexual problems become a significant concern in the situation of

---

[*] Corresponding Author's Email: suprakashch@gmail.com.

management effectiveness, as antidepressants are useful only as long as the patient takes them regularly. Unbearable adverse effects can be one reason that patients do not take medicines or stop them abruptly. However, most of the studies of drug induced sexual dysfunctions have combined data together for both males and females, barring a few. The implications of the findings will create more awareness and a better understanding of this condition and lead to effective treatment and enhancement of quality of life.

Keywords: female sexual dysfunction, depression, antidepressants

INTRODUCTION

The social construct of human sexual functioning involving its taboos, regulation, and social and political impact has played a significant role in influencing several cultures of the world since prehistoric times. The citizen's duty to control his body was an important concept of male sexuality in the Roman Republic [1]."Virtue" (virtus, from vir, "man") was equated with "manliness." The counterpart virtue for female citizens was pudicitia, a form of sexual integrity that demonstrated their attractiveness and self-control [2]. Female sexuality was encouraged within marriage. In the ancient times of the Roman culture, a man was considered a "real man" if he could govern both himself and others well, and he was expected not submit to the use or pleasure of others [3].

India has had an overwhelming impact on the history of sex, from writing one of the first literatures that treated sexual intercourse as a science, to in modern times which contributed to the origin of the philosophical emphasis of new-age groups' approaches on sex. A myriad of folk tales [4], sculptures like those in Khajuraho [5] and scholarly manuscripts reveal how love and sex between women, men, gods, semi-gods and goddesses was expressed. The initial evidence of outlooks towards human sexuality derives from the ancient texts of Hinduism, Buddhism and Jainism, the first of which are perhaps the oldest remaining literature in the world. The age-old texts, the Vedas, disclose moral viewpoints on marriage, human sexuality and fertility. The most popularly known literature on human sexuality in India is the manuscripts of the Kama Sutra. These manuscripts were created for and kept by the philosopher, warrior and nobility castes, their servants and concubines, and those in certain religious orders. These people could read and write and had instruction and education. There are several diverse versions which were written in Sanskrit and were later then translated into other languages, such as Persian or Tibetan. The version of the Kama Sutra by Vatsyayana, is one of the versions which became well known and was first translated into English by Sir Richard Burton and F. F. Arbuthnot. The Kama Sutra may presently be the most commonly read secular text in the world.

METHODS

A detailed search of the medical literature was conducted and articles from 1997-2009 were studied. Search methods included MEDLINE and PubMed databases for articles in English using search words of sexual dysfunction females/women, depression and depression and female sexual dysfunction. A total of 204 articles were screened for inclusion. In addition, bibliographies of all relevant articles were searched for further publications. All articles in this review were evaluated for relevance and methodology.

THE HUMAN SEXUAL RESPONSE

According to the current working definition by the World Health Organisation [6], sexual health is: "a state of physical, emotional, mental and social well-being in relation to sexuality; it is not merely the absence of disease, dysfunction or infirmity. Sexual health requires a positive and respectful approach to sexuality and sexual relationships, as well as the possibility of having pleasurable and safe sexual experiences, free of coercion, discrimination and violence. The sexual rights of all persons must be respected, protected and fulfilled for sexual health to be achieved and retained."

The human sexual cycle can be divided into four-stages. It is a model of physiological responses to sexual stimulation [7]. The phases of the cycle are as follows: Desire, excitement phase, plateau, orgasm, and resolution. This model was first given by William H. Masters and Virginia E. Johnson in their 1966 book titled "Human Sexual Response" [8].

CLASSIFICATIONS AND DEFINITIONS OF FEMALE SEXUAL DYSFUNCTION

The tenth edition of the international classification of mental and behavioural disorders (ICD-10) uses the term sexual dysfunction to "cover the ways in which an individual is unable to participate in a sexual relationship as he or she would wish. It includes inhibition in one or more of the phases along with disturbance in subjective sense of pleasure or desire or in the objective performance."

According to the DSM-5(The Diagnostic and Statistical Manual of Mental Disorders, fifth edition), sexual dysfunction requires a person to feel extreme distress and interpersonal strain for a minimum of 6 months (excluding substance or medication-induced sexual dysfunction) [9].

It is divides sexual dysfunction into the following categories:

- Delayed Ejaculation
- Erectile Disorder
- Female Orgasmic Disorder
- Female Sexual Interest/Arousal Disorder
- Genito-Pelvic Pain/Penetration Disorder
- Male Hypoactive Sexual Desire Disorder
- Premature (Early) Ejaculation
- Substance/Medication-Induced Sexual Dysfunction

- Other Specified Sexual Dysfunction
- Unspecified Sexual Dysfunction.

1998 AFUD CONSENSUS CLASSIFICATION OF WOMEN'S SEXUAL DISORDERS AND DYSFUNCTIONS

The American Foundation for Urologic Diseases has the following categories of female sexual dysfunction:

1. Sexual desire disorders
    A. Hypoactive sexual desire disorder
    B. Sexual aversion disorder
2. Sexual arousal disorder
3. Orgasmic disorder
4. Sexual pain disorders
    A. Dyspareunia
    B. Vaginismus
    C. Other sexual pain disorders

They are described in detail as follows:

Hypoactive Sexual Desire Disorder

Hypoactive sexual desire disorder can be defined as a persistent or recurring deficiency (or absence) of sexual fantasies/ thoughts and/or receptivity to sexual activity, which causes personal distress. It includes the following under its subheading- Sexual aversion disorder: which is a persistent or recurring phobic aversion to sexual activity and involves an active avoidance of sexual contact with a sexual partner, which may cause personal distress.

Hypoactive sexual desire disorder may result from psychological/emotional factors or be secondary to physiological problems such as hormonal deficiencies and medical or surgical interventions. A disturbance of the hormonal functioning in the females which can be caused by natural menopause, surgically or medically induced menopause, or endocrine disorders can result in inhibited sexual desire. Sexual aversion disorder is generally a psychologically or emotionally based problem that can result from a variety of causes such as physical or sexual abuse or childhood trauma.

Sexual Arousal Disorder

Sexual arousal disorder is persistent or recurring inability to attain, or maintain, sufficient sexual excitement, causing personal distress. It may be experienced as lack of subjective excitement or a lack of genital (lubrication/swelling) or other somatic responses. Sexual arousal disorders include: lack of or decreased vaginal lubrication, diminished clitoral and labial sensation, reduced clitoral and labial engorgement, and insufficient vaginal smooth muscle relaxation. These conditions can occur secondary to psychological problems or can be due to medical/physiologic causes.

Orgasmic Disorder

Orgasmic disorder is persistent or recurrent difficulty, delay in, or absence of attaining orgasm after sufficient sexual stimulation and arousal, which causes personal distress. This may be a primary (never achieved orgasm) or secondary condition, as a result of surgery, trauma, or hormonal deficiencies. Primary anorgasmia can be secondary to emotional trauma or sexual abuse; however, medical/physical factors can certainly contribute to the problem.

Sexual Pain Disorders

1. *Dyspareunia*: recurrent or persistent genital pain associated with sexual intercourse.
2. *Vaginismus*: recurrent or persistent involuntary spasm of the musculature of the outer third of the vagina that interferes with vaginal penetration, which causes personal distress.
3. *Other sexual pain disorders*: recurrent or persistent genital pain induced by noncoital sexual stimulation.

Dyspareunia can develop secondary to medical problems such as vestibulitis, vaginal atrophy, or vaginal infection; can be either physiologically or psychologically based; or can be a combination of the two. Vaginismus generally occurs as a conditioned response to painful penetration or can be secondary to psychological/emotional causes.

EPIDEMIOLOGY OF SEXUAL DYSFUNCTION IN FEMALES

Lauman et al. [10] reported the prevalence of the types of sexual dysfunction in females as follows: "a low sexual desire -22%, arousal problems 14%, and sexual pain -7% whereas in men the prevalence were as follows: premature ejaculation-21%, erectile dysfunction-5% and low sexual desire-5%." Montejo et al. [11] found that women experienced greater intensity of low libido, delayed orgasm and anorgasmia as compared to men. The most common sexual problems in females are desire and arousal dysfunctions as mentioned by McCabe et al. [12]. In addition, they stated that there are a large proportion of women who experience multiple sexual dysfunctions.

Berman et al. [13] noted that female sexual dysfunction is age-related and progressive. The aetiology of female sexual dysfunction is multifactorial. A woman's sexual dysfunction may be caused to some degree by genetics, but is influenced more by unique biological, psychological or other environmental factors [14]. The psychological causes include psychiatric illness, particularly anxiety and depression, pathological states such as vascular disease, diabetes, neurological disease and pharmacological effects of drugs can also lead to sexual dysfunction. It has long been recognised that certain antihypertensive agents, notably centrally acting sympatholytic agents, beta antagonists, and diuretics, have an adverse effect on sexual functioning [15]. Antidepressants, antipsychotics, anticonvulsants, drugs with antimuscarinic effects, steroids, proton pump inhibitors, histamine receptor blockers and chemotherapeutic agents have also been implicated [16]. The risk of having sexual problems may increase with increasing age, improper physical health, smoking more than 6 to 20 cigarettes daily, frequent use of recreational drugs including alcohol and opioid etc., loss of or low income and disturbing earlier sexual experiences [17].

DEPRESSION AND SEXUAL DYSFUNCTION

Depression is described by lack of interest in pleasurable activities, decline in energy, reduced self-esteem. Social withdrawal may impair ability to maintain intimate relationships in such people. All the above constellation of symptoms may be expected to produce difficulties in sexual relationships. Research shows that depression is connected with deficiencies of sexual function and satisfaction [18]. Kennedy et al. found that 49% of women and 26% of men with depression reported no sexual activity in preceding month [19]. Depression was found as a risk factor for sexual dysfunction in women [20]. A recent review from 2012 measured the bidirectional association of depression and sexual dysfunction, which confirmed that depression increased the risk of sexual problems and that people having sexual dysfunction had increased chances of depression [21]. The specific type of sexual dysfunction may vary in incidence, but loss of sexual desire may be more common than disorders of arousal and orgasm. In a comparative study, changes in libido were significantly more common in depressed patients than controls, but differences in the prevalence of impotence, orgasmic or ejaculatory problems were not [22].

While loss of libido is often described, problems with arousal, causing vaginal dryness, absent or delayed orgasm are also found [23]. Contrariwise, loss of sexual desire may be the reporting complaints of some patients, who after directly questioning have significant depression. In some others, loss of sexual desire may come before the onset of depression [24].

From a patho-physiological perspective, a significant percentage of depressed patients exhibit overactivity of the autonomic system and dysregulation of the neuroendocrine hypothalamic-pituitary-adrenal (HPA) axis. This is accompanied by changes in corticotropin-releasing hormone (CRH), adrenocorticotropic hormone (ACTH), beta-endorphins and catecholamines, which could increase the risks for sexual dysfunction [25] [26].

Depression and its effects on sexual functioning hamper the quality of life and should be taken into account so that treatment is holistic and complete. Asking and evaluating about sexual dysfunction will lead to proper treatment and recovery of the patients.

ANTIDEPRESSANTS AND SEXUAL DYSFUNCTION

The epidemiology of medication-induced sexual problems has been a difficult issue, due to confounding factors like mental illness, cultural influences and co-morbidity [27]. According to the DSM-5, in individuals with substance/medication-induced sexual dysfunction the disturbance in sexual function causes significant distress. Substance-induced sexual dysfunction is usually generalized and is not limited to certain types of stimulation, situations, or partners. The disturbance in sexual function should have been developed in the course of, or shortly after (within 30 days, DSM-IV-TR), substance intoxication, or after withdrawal from or exposure to a medication that may cause a problem in sexual functioning.

In the 1960s and 1970s, sporadic cases appeared in the literature oftricyclic antidepressant (TCA) and monoamine oxidase inhibitor (MAOI)induced erectile dysfunction, anorgasmia and retrograde ejaculation [28, 29]. The attention was more focused on the problem of antidepressant-induced sexual dysfunction after the introduction of Selective Serotonin Reuptake Inhibitors (SSRIs) in the latter half of the 1980s. These agents were used in a widespread manner and became famous as the first-line medicines to treat depression which further highlighted their adverse effects on sexual functioning, and threw light on their negative impact on patients' quality of life (QOL) [30].

Assessments of sexual dysfunction with SSRIs may vary, fluctuating from minor percentages to around 80% [4]. The exact occurrence is not known, and the issue is somewhat confounded by the fact that some studies report incidence and some report prevalence. Montgomery and colleagues [31] pointed out numerous obstacles to establishing the exact prevalence of antidepressant related sexual dysfunction. The data on the prevalence of sexual dysfunction is scarce, which makes it difficult to establish a normal baseline [32]. Patients with various mental disorders have an elevated risk of sexual dysfunction because of the effect of the illness on the relationships and behaviour [33]. The human sexual behaviour is subject to social and cultural influences, which may vary with time, place, ethnic group, social class etc. the data on sexual behaviour are prone to underreporting; spontaneous reporting by patients and direct questioning by physicians have been reported to differ as much as 60% [34].

Majority of studies on sexual dysfunction associated with antidepressants have methodological flaws, such as failure to use validated rating scales, a baseline assessment, a placebo group, randomization or binding. Also the reasons for the increased reporting are not entirely clear, although the trend is very likely multifactorial. Possible reasons include a much wider and more liberal use of the newer antidepressants for the other conditions; pharmacotherapy of less severe depression that was previously more likely to be treated with psychotherapy; a more sophisticated approach to evaluation of side effects; a greater emphasis on patients' quality of life and even marketing competition among pharmaceutical companies.

Sexual dysfunction is also recognized as a potential side effect of all classes of antidepressants like MAO-Inhibitors, Tricyclic antidepressants, SSRIs (Selective Serotonin Reuptake Inhibitors) and newer antidepressants) [35]. Since the launch of Selective Serotonin Reuptake Inhibitors in the market, sexual dysfunctions linked with these medications has been mentioned in efficacy studies and discussed in critical reviews [36]. The mechanism of SSRI induced sexual dysfunction is thought to involve indiscriminate stimulation of postsynaptic 5HT-2a and 5HT-2c receptors by the increased synaptic levels of serotonin [37]. Antidepressant drugs that antagonise this particular serotonin receptor subtypes like mirtazapine, nefazodone and agomelatine, have a lower chance to cause sexual problems. The reversible inhibitor of monoamine oxidase namely moclobemide, was found to increase sexual arousal and has a very low incidence of sexual dysfunction, while noradrenaline reuptake inhibitor, reboxetine, and noradrenaline and dopamine reuptake inhibitor, bupropion, have little or no effect on sexual functioning. The prior history of antidepressant-induced sexual dysfunction in a patient increases the risk of developing it again if given similar antidepressants [38].

A study done by Modell [39] found that: 73% of the patients treated with SSRI had sexual side effects compared to only 14% of patients treated with bupropion. It was found that around 77% of patients treated with bupropion reported at least one aspect of heightened sexual functioning. In a study Piazza et al. [40] suggested that after SSRI treatment, difficulties with desire and psychological arousal in depressed women tend to remit. Sexual libido and arousal problems are commonly described, though the precise correlation with SSRI use has not been regularly reported [41]. Most of the studies which have evaluated sexual dysfunction in patients getting antidepressants have included mixed sample (i.e., single and married subjects), of both genders and have not assessed for other causes like psychopathology which could influence sexual dysfunction while receiving antidepressants [42, 43, 44].

NEUROTRANSMITTERS AND SEXUAL DYSFUNCTIONS IN DEPRESSED FEMALES

Although aetiology of depression is not clear, dysregulation of neurotransmitters plays a central role. Estrogen is a known regulator of serotonin function [45]. This estrogen-serotonin interaction may explain why women exhibit higher prevalence rate of depression than men and why changes in oestrogen levels across female life cycle i.e., menopause, post-partum are associated with increased susceptibility of depression. In fact, longitudinal studies indicate that menopause transition is associated with increased risk for onset or recurrence of depressive symptoms.

Female sexual function is controlled by a multifaceted interplay between the hypophyseal-pituitary-adrenal (HPA) axis, the autonomic nervous system, circulating sex hormones i.e., testosterone, oestrogens and progesterones, neurotransmitters like serotonin, dopamine, noradrenaline, GABA and acetylcholine and vasoactive peptides such as nitric oxide [46].

Oestrogen, testosterone and progesterone promote sexual desire. Dopamine promotes desire and arousal. Norepinephrine promotes arousal. Prolactin inhibits arousal and oxytocin promotes orgasm. Prolactin's function might be to prevent arousal and studies show that serotonin decreases desire and arousal, probably by indirect means like by inhibiting noradrenaline and dopamine as well as by influencing peripheral effects of decreasing sensation, and inhibiting the vasodilator, nitric oxide. It may therefore have a function in the resolution phase of the sexual cycle [47]. Serotonin also appears to exert a peripheral effect on sexual functioning by decreasing sensation and by inhibiting nitric oxide. The serotonergic system consequently can play a role in various sexual problems [48, 49]. Vaginal NO synthase, the enzyme responsible for the production of NO, is also regulated by estrogen. Aging and surgical castration results in decreased vaginal NO levels and increased vaginal wall fibrosis [50]. Estrogen replacement restores vaginal mucosa, increases vaginal NO levels, and decreases vaginal mucosal cell death [51].

There is evidence that melatonin agonism [52] and 5-HT2C antagonism [53, 54] both favourably influence sexual behaviour.

AETIOLOGY OF FEMALE SEXUAL DYSFUNCTION

Vascular

High blood pressure, high cholesterol levels, diabetes, smoking, and heart disease are risk factors for sexual dysfunction. Similar to Leriche's syndrome in men, secondary to aortoiliac disease, clitoral and vaginal vascular insufficiency syndrome [55] results in decreased hypogastric/ pudendal arterial bed in women, resulting in decreased inflow to the clitoris or vagina. This is primarily due to atherosclerosis of the iliohypogastric/ pudendal arterial bed. Reduced pelvic blood flow resulting from aortoiliac or atherosclerotic disease causes vaginal wall and clitoral smooth muscle fibrosis [56]. Histological examination of clitoral erectile tissue from atherosclerotic animals demonstrated cavernosal artery wall thickening, loss of corporal smooth muscle, and increases in collagen deposition. In human clitoral tissue, there is a loss of corporal smooth muscle and replacement by fibrous connective tissue in association with atherosclerosis of clitoral cavernosal arteries. Any trauma to the ilio-hypogastric pudendal arterial bed results from pelvic fractures, blunt trauma, surgical disruption, or chronic perineal pressure from bicycle riding, can result in diminished vaginal and clitoral blood flow and may lead to sexual dysfunction.

Neurological

The same neurologic disorders that cause erectile dysfunction in men can also cause sexual dysfunction in women. Spinal cord injury or disease of the central or peripheral nervous system, including diabetes, can result in neurogenic female sexual dysfunction. Women with complete upper motor neuron injuries affecting sacral spinal segments are unable to achieve psychogenic lubrication; however, women with incomplete injuries retain the capacity for psychogenic lubrication [57]. Females with spinal cord injury have notably more problem achieving orgasm [58]. The effects of specific spinal cord injuries on female sexual response is being investigated, and it is hoped will lead to improved understanding of the neurophysiology of orgasm and arousal in normal women.

Hormonal/Endocrine

Hormonally based female sexual dysfunction can be caused due to dysfunction of the hypothalamic/pituitary axis, surgical or medical castration, natural menopause, premature ovarian failure, and chronic birth control pill use. The patients usually present with complaints of decreased desire and libido, vaginal dryness, and lack of sexual arousal.

Psychological

Irrespective of the presence or absence of organic disease, emotional and relational problems considerably affect sexual arousal in women. Issues such as self-esteem, body image, relationship with her partner, and ability to communicate her sexual needs to her partner all impact sexual function. In addition, psychological disorders (e.g., depression, obsessive compulsive disorder, anxiety disorder) are associated with female sexual dysfunction.

Medications

Medications used to treat depression can also significantly affect the female sexual response. The most frequently used medications for uncomplicated depression are serotonin reuptake inhibitors. Women receiving these medications often complain of decreased sexual interest and desire, decreased arousal, decreased genital sensation, and difficulty achieving orgasm [59]. Recently, several publications have reported the successful use of sildenafil to treat SSRI-induced female sexual dysfunction [60].

TREATMENT OF SEXUAL DYSFUNCTION IN DEPRESSED FEMALES

Given the scarcity of evidence based treatments in the management of female sexual dysfunction is still an art rather than a science. Even seemingly clear-cut case of medication associated sexual dysfunction should not be treated in a strictly biological sense. The overall treatment always take into consideration psychological factors and normal fluctuation of sexual functioning. It should promote a healthy lifestyle, recommending for example weight reduction, exercise, smoking cessation and treatment of substance use.

A healthy lifestyle can be helpful in a variety of ways including enhancing self-image, sense of well-being, overall health and the health of physiological systems related to sexual response system. Some patients may have pre-treatment lifestyle related sexual dysfunctions in addition to an SSRI associated sexual dysfunction such as those caused by chronic use of alcohol or tobacco. Reducing the severity of lifestyle related sexual dysfunction may render the SSRI related sexual dysfunction more manageable.

Sexual disorders even minor ones may lead to frustration, worry and stress. They have a serious impact on the life and happiness of an individual and couple. Several strategies may be beneficial in the management of treatment associated sexual dysfunction in depression. They include behavioural techniques to improve sexual functioning, psychoeducation about myths and misconceptions etc. Another strategy includes the "drug holiday." It was described by Rothchild [61]. In this strategy the patients stop their antidepressant for several days (e.g., a weekend) in anticipation of sex. For most of the patients, this approach is successful. However, for those taking the long-half-life agent fluoxetine, it might not work. Moreover, some patients experience a reappearance of depressive symptoms during this time. Zwillich [62] expressed scepticism about this strategy. According to him, some patients may experience withdrawal effects and may encourage medication noncompliance.

Few pharmacological agents have been tried and tested for treatment. These are as follows:

1. *Flibanserin* has been approved by the U. S. Food and Drug Administration for the management of hypoactive sexual desire disorder (HSDD) of premenopausal women [63].
2. *Estrogen Replacement Therapy*: Estrogen replacement therapy is indicated in menopausal women. It not only decreases hot flashes, prevents osteoporosis, and lowers the risk of heart disease, but also results in better clitoral sensitivity, improvement in the libido, and reduced pain during intercourse. Symptoms of vaginal dryness, burning, and urinary frequency and urgency can be decreased by applying local or topical estrogen application. In menopausal women or oophorectomized women, complaints of vaginal irritation, pain, or dryness, secondary to vaginal atrophy, can be relieved with topical estrogen cream. A vaginal estradiol ring is now available that delivers low-dose estrogen locally, which may benefit patients with breast cancer and other women unable to take oral or transdermal estrogen [64].
3. *Methyl Testosterone*: Methyl testosterone is often used in combination with estrogen in menopausal women for symptoms of inhibited desire, dyspareunia, or lack of vaginal lubrication. There are conflicting reports regarding the benefit of methyl testosterone for the treatment of inhibited desire and/or vaginismus in premenopausal women. Topical testosterone cream is an approved treatment for vaginal lichen planus. Potential benefits of this therapy include increased clitoral sensitivity, increased vaginal

lubrication, increased libido, and heightened arousal. Potential side effects of testosterone administration, either topical or oral, include weight gain, clitoral enlargement, increased facial hair, and hypercholesterolemia.

4. *Sildenafil*: Functioning as a selective type V (cGMP-specific) phosphodiesterase inhibitor, sildenafil decreases catabolism of cGMP, the second messenger in NO-mediated relaxation of clitoral and vaginal smooth muscle [65]. Sildenafil can be useful when used alone or perhaps in combination with other vasoactive substances for treatment of female sexual arousal disorder. Clinical studies evaluating the safety and efficacy of this medication in women with sexual arousal disorder are currently in progress. Several studies are already published demonstrating the efficacy of sildenafil for treatment of female sexual dysfunction secondary to SSRI use [66, 67]. Another study was recently published describing the subjective effects of sildenafil in a population of postmenopausalwomen [68]. A Systematic review and meta-analysis done by Gao L et al. demonstrated that phosphodiesterase type 5 inhibitors could be an effective treatment modality for female sexual dysfunction [69].

5. *Prostaglandin E1*: An intraurethral application of prostaglandin E1, absorbed by the mucosa, is now available for male patients. A similar application of prostaglandin E1 delivered intravaginally is currently under investigation for use in women. Clinical studies are necessary to determine the efficacy of this medication in the treatment of female sexual dysfunction.

6. If a patient's depression (or other syndrome for which antidepressants are prescribed, e.g., obsessive compulsive disorder) is in good remission, but sexual functioning remains a problem, doctors often try purported antidotes. This was recently reviewed by Labbate [70]. One strategy is to employ drugs that block some serotonin receptors. Examples include the appetite-stimulating antihistamine cyproheptadine, the antimigraine methysergide, the anxiolytic buspirone, and the antidepressants

nefazodone, mirtazapine, and mianserin. The addition of bupropion at higher doses is the approach studied commonly for women with antidepressant-induced sexual dysfunction [71]. A systematic assessment of sexual function among depressed outpatients found that mirtazapine enhanced sexual functioning in both men and women [72].

7. *Dopamine Agonists*: Another strategy employs dopamine agonists on the theory that enhanced dopamine neurotransmission appears to promote some aspects of sexual function. Examples include amantadine, amphetamine, and methylphenidate.
8. *Yohimbine*, an adrenergic antagonist with purported aphrodisiac effects, is sometimes employed as a presumed sexual antidote.
9. The herbal preparation *ginkgo biloba*, recently reported to be effective in reversing memory difficulties in the elderly, has been claimed to enhance sexual function. Anecdotal reports suggest it might play a role in reversing dysfunction due to antidepressants [73].

Follow-up is extremely important, regardless of the treatment option. Keep an eye out for adverse effects, evaluating satisfaction or outcome of the given treatment, establishing if the partner is suffering from a sexual dysfunction also, and keeping in mind that the overall health and psychosocial function are important aspects of follow-up [74, 75].

CONCLUSION

Women being reticent about sex may not report with sexual problems unless specific enquiry is made about the same. This highlights the fact that we should be extremely vigilant with females presenting to our clinics with depression and should regularly ask them for sexual problems as they may not tell it themselves even if the problem is present.

REFERENCES

[1] McGinn, T. A. J. (1998). *Prostitution, Sexuality and the Law in Ancient Rome*. New York: Oxford University Press.

[2] Langlands, R. (2006). *Sexual Morality in Ancient Rome*. Cambridge: Cambridge University Press.

[3] Cantarella, E. (1992). *Bisexuality in the Ancient World*. New Haven: Yale University Press.

[4] Pattanaik, D. (2002). *The Man Who Was A Woman And Other Queer Tales of Hindu lore*. Philadelphia: Routledge.

[5] Allen, James A. (1999) The Mystery of the Smiling Elephant: In the Erotic Temples of Khajuraho. *The Georgia Review* 53(2), 321–340.

[6] World Health Organization. (2010). *Measuring sexual health: conceptual and practical considerations and related indicators*. Geneva: WHO.

[7] Archer, J., and Lloyd, B. (2002). *Sex and Gender*. Cambridge: Cambridge University Press.

[8] Masters, W. H., and Johnson, V. E. (1981) *Human Sexual Response*. New York: Bantam.

[9] Nolen-Hoeksema, S. (2014). *Abnormal Psychology*. New York: McGraw-Hill.

[10] Laumann, E., Paik, A., and Rosen, R. C. (1999). Sexual dysfunction in the United States: prevalence and predictors. *JAMA* 281(6), 537-544.

[11] Montejo, A. L., Llorca, G., Tzquierdo, J. A., and Rico-Vilademoros, F. (2001). Incidence of sexual dysfunction associated with antidepressant agents: A prospective multi-centre study of 1022 outpatients. *Journal of Clinical Psychiatry* 62, 10-22.

[12] McCabe, M. P., Sharlip, I. D., Lewis, R., Atalla, E., Balon, R., Fisher, A. D., Laumann, E., Lee, S. W., and Segraves, R. T. (2016). Incidence and Prevalence of Sexual Dysfunction in Women and Men: A Consensus Statement from the Fourth International Consultation on Sexual Medicine 2015. *Journal of Sexual Medicine* 13(2), 144-152.

[13] Berman, J. R., Berman, L., and Goldstein, A. I. (1999). Female sexual dysfunction: Incidence, pathophysiology, evaluation and treatment options. *Urology* 54, 385-391.
[14] Clayton, A., and Groth, J. (2013). Etiology of Female Sexual Dysfunction. *Women's Health* 9(2), 135-137.
[15] Ellison, K. E., and Gandhi, G. (2005). Optimising the use of β-adrenoceptor antagonists in coronary artery disease. *Drugs* 65(6), 787–797.
[16] Yang, B., and Donatucci, C. (2006) Drugs that affect male sexual function. In: Mulcahy JJ, Totowa NJ (eds). *Current clinical urology: male sexual function: a guide to clinical management.* 2nd edition. New York: Springer.
[17] Clayton, A. H., Pradko, J., and Croft, H. (2002). Prevalence of sexual dysfunction among newer antidepressants. *Journal of Clinical Psychiatry* 63, 357–366.
[18] Baldwin, D. (2001). Depression and sexual dysfunction. *British Medical Bulletin* 57(1), 81-99.
[19] Kennedy, S., Dickens, S., Eisfeld, B., and Bagby, R. (1999) Sexual dysfunction before antidepressant therapy in major depression. *Journal of Affective Disorders* 56(2-3), 201-208.
[20] Zieba, A., Dudek, D., Jawor, M., and Krzysiek, J. (1998). Sexual dysfunctions in depressed patients. *Psychiatria Polska* 32(5), 621-628.
[21] Atlantis, E., and Sullivan, T. (2012). Bidirectional Association between Depression and Sexual Dysfunction: A Systematic Review and Meta-Analysis. *The Journal of Sexual Medicine* 9(6), 1497-1507.
[22] Mathew, R., and Weinman, M. (1982). Sexual dysfunctions in depression. *Archives of Sexual Behavior* 11(4), 323-328.
[23] Kennedy, S., and Rizvi, S. (2009). Sexual Dysfunction, Depression, and the Impact of Antidepressants. *Journal of Clinical Psychopharmacology* 29(2), 157-164.
[24] Schreiner-Engel, P., and Schiavi, R. (1986). Lifetime Psychopathology in Individuals with Low Sexual Desire. *The Journal of Nervous and Mental Disease* 174(11):646-651.

[25] Goldstein, I. (2000). The mutually reinforcing triad of depressive symptoms, cardiovascular disease and erectile dysfunction. *American Journal of Cardiology* 86, 41F–44F.

[26] Rosen, R. C., Lane, R., and Menza, M. (1999). Effects of SSRI on sexual dysfunction: a critical review. *Journal of Clinical Psychopharmacology* 19: 67–71.

[27] Balon, R. (2006). SSRI-associated sexual dysfunction. *American Journal of Psychiatry* 163, 1504–1509.

[28] Monteiro, W. O., Noshirvani, H. F., and Marks, I. M. (1987). Anorgasmia from clomipramine in obsessional compulsive disorder: a controlled trial. *British Journal of Psychiatry* 151, 107–112.

[29] Segraves, R. T. (1993). Treatment emergent sexual dysfunction in affective disorder: a review and management strategies. *Journal of Clinical Psychiatry Monograph* 11, 57–63.

[30] Baldwin, D. S. (2004). Sexual dysfunction associated with antidepressant drugs. *Expert Opinion Drug Safety* 3, 457–470.

[31] Montgomery, S. (2002). Antidepressant medications: a review of the evidence for drug-induced sexual dysfunction. *Journal of Affective Disorders* 69(1-3), 119-140.

[32] Laumann, E., Nicolosi, A., Glasser, D., Paik, A., Gingell, C., Moreira, E. et al. (2004). Sexual problems among women and men aged 40–80 y: prevalence and correlates identified in the Global Study of Sexual Attitudes and Behaviors. *International Journal of Impotence Research* 17(1), 39-57.

[33] Casper, R. (1985). Somatic Symptoms in Primary Affective Disorder. *Archives of General Psychiatry* 42(11), 1098.

[34] Montejo-González, A. L., Llorca, G., Izquierdo, J. A., Ledesma, A., Bousoño, M., Calcedo, A., Carrasco, J. L., Ciudad, J., Daniel, E., De la Gandara, J., Derecho, J., Franco, M., Gomez, M. J., Macias, J. A., Martin, T., Perez, V., Sanchez, J. M., Sanchez, S., and Vicens, E. (1997). SSRI-induced sexual dysfunction: fluoxetine, paroxetine, sertraline, and fluvoxamine in a prospective, multicenter, and descriptive clinical study of 344 patients. *Journal of Sex & Marital Therapy* 23(3), 176-194.

[35] Montgomery, S. A., Baldwin, D. S., and Riley, A. (2002) Antidepressant medications: A review of the evidence for drug-induced sexual dysfunction. *Journal of Affective Disorders* 2002; 69:119-40.

[36] Rosen, R., Lane, R., and Menza, M. (1999). Effects of SSRIs on Sexual Function. *Journal of Clinical Psychopharmacology* 19(1), 67-85.

[37] Mir, S., and Taylor, D. (1998). Sexual adverse effects with new antidepressants. *Psychiatric Bulletin* 22, 438–441.

[38] Clayton, A. H., and Montejo, A. L. (2006). Major depressive disorder, antidepressants, and sexual dysfunction. *Journal of Clinical Psychiatry* 67(6), 33–37.

[39] Modell, J. G., Katholi, C. R., Modell, J. D., and DePalma, R. L. (1997). Comparative sexual side effects of bupropion, fluoxetine, paroxetine, and sertraline. *Clinical Pharmacology and Therapeutics* 61(4), 476-487.

[40] Piazza, L. A., Markowitz, J. C., Kocsis, J. H., Leon, A. C., Portera, L., Miller, N. L., and Adler, D. (1997). Sexual functioning in chronically depressed patients treated with SSRI antidepressants: a pilot study. *American Journal of Psychiatry* 154(12), 1757-1759.

[41] Mathew, R., and Weinman, M. (1982). Sexual dysfunctions in depression. *Archives of Sexual Behavior* 11(4), 323-328.

[42] Moreira, E. D., Glasser, D. B., Nicolosi, A., Duarte, F. G., Gingell, C., and GSSAB Investigators' Group. (2008). Sexual problems and help-seeking behaviour in adults in the United Kingdom and continental Europe. *British Journal of Urology International* 101, 1005-1011.

[43] Pollack, M. H., Reiter, S, and Hammerness, P. (1992) Genitourinary and sexual adverse effects of psychotropic medication. *International Journal of Psychiatry in Medicine* 22, 305-327.

[44] Delgado, P., Brannan, S., Mallinckrodt, C., Tran, P. V., McNamara, R. K., Wang, F., et al. (2005). Sexual functioning assessed in 4 double-blind placebo- and paroxetine-controlled trials of duloxetine

for major depressive disorder. *Journal of Clinical Psychiatry* 66, 686-692.

[45] Lu, N. (2002). Ovarian Steroid Regulation of 5-HT1A Receptor Binding and G protein Activation in Female Monkeys. *Neuropsychopharmacology* 27(1):12-24.

[46] Raina, R. (2007). Female sexual dysfunction: classification, pathophysiology, and management. *Fertility and Sterility* 88(5), 1273–1284.

[47] Meston, C. M., and Frohlich, P. F. (2002). The neurobiology of sexual function. *Arch Gen Psychiatry* 57, 1012–30.

[48] Clayton, A. (2003). Sexual function and dysfunction in women. *Psychiatric Clinics of North America* 26(3), 673-682.

[49] Levin, R. (1992). The Mechanisms of Human Female Sexual Arousal. *Annual Review of Sex Research* 3(1), 1-48.

[50] Berman, J., McCarthy, M, and Kyprianou, N. (1998). Effect of estrogen withdrawal on nitric oxide synthase expression and apoptosis in the rat vagina. *Urology* 44, 650–656.

[51] Ottesen, B., Ulrichsen, H., Frahenkrug, J., Larsen, J. J., Wagner, G., Schierup, L., and Søndergaard, F. (1982). Vasoactive intestinal polypeptide and the female genital tract: relationship to reproductive phase and delivery. *American Journal of Obstetrics and Gynecology* 43: 414–420.

[52] Drago, F., and Busa, L. (2000). Acute low doses of melatonin restore full sexual activity in impotent male rats. *Brain Research* 878, 98–104.

[53] Hull, E. M., Muschamp, J. W., and Sato, S. (2004). Dopamine and serotonin: influences on male sexual behaviour. *Physiology and Behavior* 83, 291–307.

[54] Klint, T., and Larsson, K. (1995). Clozapine acts as a 5HT2 antagonist by attenuating DOI-induced inhibition of male rat sexual behaviour. *Psychopharmacology* 119: 291–294.

[55] Myers, L. S., and Morokof, P. J. (1986). Physiological and subjective sexual arousal in pre- and postmenopausal women taking replacement therapy. *Psychophysiology* 23, 283.

[56] Park, K., Goldstein, I., Andry, C., Siroky, M. B., Krane, R. J., Azadzoi, K. M. (1997). Vasculogenic female sexual dysfunction: the hemodynamic basis for vaginal en-gorgement insufficiency and clitoral erectile insufficiency. *International Journal of Impotence Research* 9, 27–37.

[57] Tarcan, T., Park, K., Goldstein, I., Maio, G., Fassina, A., Krane, R. J., and Azadzoi, K. M. (1999). Histomorphometric analysis of age-related structural changes in human clitoral cavernosal tissue. *Journal of Urology* 161, 940–943.

[58] Sipski, M. L., Alexander, C. J., and Rosen, R. C. (1999). Sexual response in women with spinal cord injuries: implications for our understanding of the able-bodied. *Journal of Sex and Marital Therapy* 25, 11–22.

[59] Weiner, D. N., and Rosen, R. C. (1997). Medications and their impact. In Colilla J (Ed). *Sexual Function in People with Disability and Chronic Illness: A Health Professionals Guide*. Gaithersburg, Maryland, Aspen Publications. pp 85–115.

[60] Nurnberg, H. G., Lodillo, J., Hensley, P., Parker, L. M., and Keith, S. J. (1999). Sildenafil for iatrogenic seratonergic antidepressant medication-induced sexual dysfunction in 4 patients. *Journal of Clinical Psychiatry* 60, 33–38.

[61] Rothschild, A. J. (1995). Selective serotonin reuptake inhibitor-induced sexual dysfunction: efficacy of a drug holiday. *American Journal of Psychiatry* 152, 1514–1516.

[62] Zwillich, T. (1999). Beware of long-term effects of antidepressants. *Clinical Psychiatry News* 9, 16.

[63] Sang, J. H., Kim, T. H., Kim, S. A. (2016). Flibanserin for Treating Hypoactive Sexual Desire Disorder. *Journal of Menopausal Medicine* 22(1), 9-13.

[64] Ayton, R. A., Darting, G. M., Murkies, A. L., Farrell, E. A., Weisberg, E., Selinus, I. and Fraser, I. S. (1996). A comparative study of safety and efficacy of continuous low dose estradiol released from a vaginal ring compared with conjugated equine estrogen

vaginal cream in the treatment of postmenopausal vaginal atrophy. *British Journal of Obstetrics and Gynaecology* 103: 351–358.

[65] Goldstein, I., and Berman, J. R. (1998). Vasculogenic female sexual dysfunction: vaginal engorgement and clitoral erectile insufficiency syndromes. *International Journal of Impotence Research* 10, S84 – S90.

[66] Sipski, M. L., Alexander, C. J., and Rosen R. C. (1999). Sexual response in women with spinal cord injuries: implications for our understanding of the able-bodied. *Journal of Sex and Marital Therapy* 25, 11–22.

[67] Laan, E., and Everaerd, W. (1998). Physiological measures of vaginal vasocongestion. *International Journal of Impotence Research* 10, S107–S110.

[68] Kaplan SA, Rodolfo RB, Kohn IJ, Ikeguchi, I. F., Laor, E., and Te A. E. (1999). Safety and efficacy of sildenafil in postmenopausal women with sexual dysfunction. *Urology* 53: 481–486.

[69] Gao L, Yang L, Qian S, Li T, Han P, and Yuan J. (2016). Systematic review and meta-analysis of phosphodiesterase type 5 inhibitors for the treatment of female sexual dysfunction. *International Journal of Gynaecology and Obstetrics* 133(2), 139-45.

[70] Labbate, L. A. (1999). Sex and serotonin reuptake inhibitor antidepressants. *Psychiatric Clinics of North America* 29, 571–579.

[71] Taylor M, Rudkin L, and Hawton K. (2005). Strategies for managing antidepressant-induced sexual dysfunction: Systematic review of randomised controlled trials. *Journal of Affective Disorders* 88(3), 241-254.

[72] Boyarsky BK, Haque W, Rouleau MR, and Hirschfeld RM. (1999). Sexual functioning in depressed outpatients taking mirtazapine. *Depression Anxiety* 9, 175–179.

[73] Cohen, A. J., and Bartlik, B. (1998). Gingko biloba for antidepressant induced sexual dysfunction. *Journal of Sex and Marital Therapy* 24, 139–143.

[74] Atiemo, H. O., Szostak, M. J., and Sklar, G. N. (2003). Salvage of sildenafil failures referred from primary care physicians. *Journal of Urology* 170, 2356–2358.

[75] Souverein, P. C., Egberts, A. C., Meuleman, E. J., Urquhart, J., and Leufkens, H. G. (2002). Incidence and determinants of sildenafil (dis)continuation: The Dutch cohort of sildenafil users. *International Journal of Impotence Research* 2002;14:259–65.

In: Depression and Anxiety
Editor: Shelley L. Becker

ISBN: 978-1-53617-229-4
© 2020 Nova Science Publishers, Inc.

Chapter 3

A COMPARATIVE STUDY OF THE USE OF BENZODIAZEPINES AMONG PATIENTS WITH MAJOR DEPRESSION AND ANXIETY DISORDERS

María Yoldi-Negrete[1], Rebeca Robles-García[2], Nicolás Martínez-López[1], Sara Martínez-Camarillo[3], Mariana Jiménez-Tirado[3], Carlos-Alfonso Tovilla-Zárate[4], Eduardo Madrigal[5] and Ana Fresán[1],*

[1]Subdirección de Investigaciones Clínicas. Instituto Nacional de Psiquiatría Ramón de la Fuente Muñíz, Ciudad de México, Mexico
[2]Centro de Investigación en Salud Mental Global, Instituto Nacional de Psiquiatría Ramón de la Fuente Muñíz, Ciudad de México, Mexico
[3]Clínica de Trastornos Afectivos. Instituto Nacional de Psiquiatría Ramón de la Fuente Muñíz, Ciudad de México, Mexico
[4]Universidad Juárez Autónoma de Tabasco, División Académica Multidisciplinaria de Comalcalco, Comalcalco, Tabasco, Mexico

---

* Corresponding Author's Email: fresan@imp.edu.mx; a_fresan@yahoo.com.mx.

[5]Dirección General, Instituto Nacional de Psiquiatría Ramón de la Fuente Muñíz, Ciudad de México, Mexico

Abstract

Introduction. Benzodiazepines (BZDs) are some of the most frequently prescribed psychotropic medications in the world. Under proper prescription, BZDs have sedative and antianxiety properties useful for specific purposes in the treatment of several mental conditions, such as anxiety disorders and depression. For depression, BZDs are not routinely indicated due to their lack of antidepressant effect, but their short-term use may be helpful when depression displays severe anxiety symptoms. In general, as stated in several clinical guidelines and expert consensus, it is recommended the short-term use of BZDs and a continuous clinical monitoring of their use, as the long-term use may be associated to several complications, including dependence and worsening of the underlying condition.

The present study aims to contribute to the body of knowledge about BZDs use in middle-income countries, such as Mexico, where an important number of patients with anxiety disorders and depression are treated for prolonged periods with BZDs. Therefore, the objective was to compare BZD use between patients with major depression and anxiety disorders (generalized anxiety disorder and panic disorder) to determine which demographic features are related to BZD use and constitute risk factors for BZD dependence.

We hypothesize that both groups will report a prolonged time of BZDs use, and more patients with anxiety disorders will exhibit BZD dependence; while being a woman, having an older age, being single, with a more prolonged use of BZDs and having an anxiety disorder will be risk factors for BZD dependence.

Method. A total of 158 patients were recruited from the outpatient service at a highly specialized psychiatric facility in Mexico City. Patients were included if they were over 18 years of age and met DSM-IV criteria for major depression, generalized anxiety disorder or panic disorder without any other significant comorbidity and were current BZDs users.

Diagnosis of major depression and anxiety disorders (generalized anxiety disorder and panic disorder) were determined with the Structured Clinical Interview for DSM-IV Axis I Disorders (SCID-I). Also, to determine BZD dependence, an adapted version of the substance dependence section of the SCID-I designed to assess BZD use exclusively was used. Demographic features and characteristics of BZD use of each patients were obtained by a face-to-face interview with the patient. To assess the subjective experience with BZDs in the last month, the Benzodiazepine Dependence Questionnaire in its Mexican version (BDEPQ-MX) was used.

For the comparison between groups chi square tests and independent samples t Tests were used while two multivariate logistic regression models with the backward conditional method were used to determine risk factors associated to BZD dependence in patients with depression and anxiety disorders.

Results. From the patients included, 55.7% (n = 88) had an anxiety disorder and the remaining 44.3% (n = 70) were diagnosed with major depression. Women accounted for most patients with depression (82.9% vs. 69.3%) while patients with anxiety disorders were younger (50.4 vs. 56.1 years). Patients with anxiety disorders had an earlier onset of BZD use (39.7 vs. 46.6 years). Insomnia, as the main reason for BZD use was reported in 47.1% (n = 33) of patients with depression and only in 20.5% (n = 18) of patients with anxiety disorders. BZD dependence was more frequently observed in patients with anxiety disorders (58.0% vs. 41.4%). No differences between groups were observed in terms of the subjective experience with BZD assessed with the BDEPQ-MX. Time of consumption was over 7 years for both groups.

The results of the logistic regression models showed that time of consumption was a risk factor for BZD dependence in both groups, while protective factors for BZD dependence included being a male in patients with anxiety disorders, and being younger for patients with depression

Discussion. In present study, several differences between patients with major depression and anxiety disorders related to BZD use were found. Long-term use of BZDs was observed in both groups and was the main predictor for BZD dependence. Although the presence of anxious symptoms was the most frequent reason for BZD prescription, an important percentage of patients with depression use these medications for insomnia, which may expose the patients to several risks associated to BZD use.

Safety and efficacy of the long-term use of BZD has been subject of controversy. Restriction in prescription may also be ineffective as BZDs may be prescribed repeatedly, resulting in long-term use.

Further studies assessing safety and effectiveness, as well as efforts to encourage and train clinicians and patients to use other alternative medications and non-pharmacological interventions for symptoms where BZDs are prescribed, such as anxiety and insomnia, are necessary to develop complementary treatments without the clinical risks associated to BZDs use.

Although the effectivity of BZDs has been proved, clinicians and patients should establish clear and specific goals for their use since the initial treatment plan for depression and anxiety disorders.

Keywords: benzodiazepine use, depression, anxiety, dependence

INTRODUCTION

Benzodiazepines (BZD) are some of the most frequently prescribed psychotropic medications in the everyday clinical practice (Fang et al. 2009; Fassaert et al. 2007; Greenblatt, Harmatz, and Shader 2018; Moylan et al. 2011; Ciuna et al. 2004). BZD use in Mexico is in accordance to that described in other countries: they represent the most prescribed drugs consumed by the population (Villatoro et al. 2012; Minaya et al. 2011).

BZD in general have sedative effects, antiepileptic effects, anxiolytic effects and effects on memory; they are therefore approved for insomnia, anxiety and panic disorders, epileptic syndromes, skeletal muscle spasms and alcohol withdrawal (Howard et al. 2014). Their effect on anxiety symptoms is widely recognized and safe for the short-term use[1]. Clinical guidelines state that "benzodiazepine doses should be as low as possible, but as high as necessary" (Bandelow et al. 2008). They are not approved for treating depression, although they are frequently administered alongside antidepressants due to the high comorbidity between depression and anxiety. Simultaneous administration of BZD and antidepressants for a brief period of time has been found to improve outcomes, most probably due to an improved tolerance to antidepressant side-effects, which are common in the first two weeks of treatment (Ogawa et al. 2019).

However, anxiety disorders and depression with comorbid anxiety, present in a chronic, waxing and waning course for which treatment should ideally be continued for at least one year after complete remission of symptoms (Bandelow et al. 2008). The continued use of BZD must be subject to careful analysis as risks may outweigh benefits when the first 90 days of treatment have elapsed.

Indeed, the long-term use of BZD has been associated with significant side-effects: dependence, withdrawal symptoms, relapse anxiety, falls and

---

[1] Short term use is defined as prescription of BZD within the first 90 days from diagnosis (Sjöstedt et al. 2017).

fractures and cognitive impairment (Crowe and Stranks 2018; Sjöstedt et al. 2017; Airagnes et al. 2019; Bandelow et al. 2008; Richardson et al. 2019). Of these, dependence is of particular importance as it increases the risk for all other side-effects as it involves a continued use.

BZD dependence has been reported in up to 44% of chronic users (O'brien 2005; Minaya et al. 2011) and even higher in certain populations such as older adults, which are, paradoxically, the most vulnerable (Minaya, Ugalde, and Fresán 2009). Given the importance of dependence to BZD, several studies have tried to determine the risk factors associated with long-term use of BZD. Age older than 65, high dosage (>5 mg diazepam per day), prescription made by a psychiatrist and BZD polytherapy are associated with higher risk. Regarding patients with depression and anxiety disorders, demographic factors related to long-term BZD use are older age, middle socioeconomic status, being on social welfare and not being married (Sjöstedt et al. 2017). In contrast, the prescription of hypnotics and concurrent use of antipsychotics or alternative drugs to BZD are associated with their discontinuation (Kanazawa et al. 2018).

However, whether risk factors for BZD dependence differ between patients with major depression and anxiety disorders (generalized anxiety disorder and panic disorder) remains unknown. Indeed, the reasons for prescribing BZD in depressed patients may vary from those leading to prescription of such agents in patients with anxiety disorders. For example, BZD might be used to treat insomnia and not necessarily anxious symptoms. Also, depressed patients are more likely to be prescribed with antidepressants than patients with anxiety disorders (Barbui et al. 2011), which represents a protective factor for long-term use and BZD misuse as previously stated: concomitant use of antidepressants and antipsychotics are associated with discontinuation of BZD (Bushnell et al. 2017; Kanazawa et al. 2018).

The present study aims to contribute to the body of knowledge about BZD use in middle-income countries, such as Mexico, where an important number of patients with anxiety disorders and depression are treated for prolonged periods with BZD. Therefore, the objective of the present study was to compare BZD use between patients with major depression and anxiety disorders (generalized anxiety disorder and panic disorder) to determine which demographic features are related to BZD use and risk factors for BZD dependence.

We hypothesize that both groups will report a prolonged time of BZD use, and more patients with anxiety disorders will exhibit BZD dependence. Being a woman, having an older age, being single, with a more prolonged use of BZD and having an anxiety disorder will be the most important factors associated to BZD dependence.

METHODS

The present study was approved by the Ethics and Research Committees of the National Institute of Psychiatry Ramón de la Fuente Muñíz (Instituto Nacional de Psiquiatría Ramón de la Fuente Muñíz – INPRFM). All patients gave their written informed consent to voluntarily participate after receiving a comprehensive explanation of the aims and procedures of the study.

Participants and Setting

All patients were recruited at the outpatient services of the INPRFM, a highly specialized mental health facility dedicated to resource training, brief and long-term treatment of psychiatric patients and research in Mexico City. The present cross-sectional study was performed by a convenience sample including patients meeting the following criteria: (a) 18 years or older, (b) met DSM-IV criteria for major depression, generalized anxiety disorder or panic disorder as the main diagnosis of current psychiatric treatment without any other significant comorbidity, (c) clinically stable according to the treating psychiatrist and medical record and (c) who were under current treatment with BZDs. Patients were excluded if they had a history of bipolar or psychotic disorder (reviewed at clinical records), current or previous substance abuse or dependence (except for BZDs) or high suicide risk or risk of agitation during the assessment.

Assessment Procedure

Diagnosis of major depression and anxiety disorders (generalized anxiety disorder and panic disorder) were firstly identified by the review of clinical charts and confirmed with the Structured Clinical Interview for DSM-IV Axis I Disorders (SCID-I) (First et al., 1996). Demographic information (sex, age, education, marital and laboral status) and BZD use features were registered in a previously design format and assessed by a face-to-face interview with each patient. BZD use features evaluated were: (1) age of first BZD prescription, (2) medical reason for BZD prescription and (3) total duration of BZD use (in weeks).

Also, an adapted version of the substance dependence section of the SCID-I designed to assess BZD dependence exclusively was used. For those patients meeting criteria for dependence, severity was registered according to clinical judgement of the clinician performing the evaluation.

To assess the subjective experience with BZDs in the last month, the Benzodiazepine Dependence Questionnaire in its Mexican version (BDEPQ-MX) (Baillie and Mattick, 1996; Minaya et al., 2011) was used. This is a self-administered 30-item questionnaire that measures BZD dependence syndrome experiences in the last month in three major subscales: (1) general dependence, (2) pleasant effects and (3) perceived need. The BDEPQ was validated for its in Mexican Psychiatric patients with adequate construct validity and internal consistency.

Statistical Analysis

For the comparison between patients with major depression and anxiety disorders chi square tests and independent samples t Tests were used. Effect sizes were computed for the significant results obtained in the Chi-square tests (Cramer's V) and the Student t-tests (Cohen d) and values were interpreted as small (0.2 – 0.3), medium (0.4 – 0.7) and large (>0.8). In addition, a multivariate logistic regression with the backward conditional method was used to determine risk factors associated to BZD dependence in these patients including demographic and BZDs use features. Significance level for all tests was established at $p < 0.05$. All statistical procedures were performed using the Statistical Package for the Social Sciences (SPSS), version 21.

RESULTS

Demographic Characteristics

A total of 158 patients with a mean age of 50.4 years (S.D. = 15.7, 19-83 years) were recruited. Women accounted for most of the patients recruited (75.3%, n = 119) and just over 50% of the sample were single (50.6%, n = 80) and dedicated to housewife activities (55.1%, n = 87) at the time of the study. Mean level of education was 10.4 years (S.D. = 4.4, range 0-19 years) and patients had a low (43.7%, n = 69) or medium (36.1%, n = 57) socioeconomic status. After the SCID-I interview, patients were grouped in those with an anxiety disorder (55.7%, n = 88; 60 with GAD and 28 with panic disorder) and the remaining 44.3% (n = 70) in the group of patients with major depression.

A higher proportion of women were found in the group of major depression (82.9% vs. 69.3%, p = 0.05, Cramer's V = 0.15), while patients with anxiety disorders were younger 50.4 years vs. 56.1 years, p = 0.02, Cohen's d = 0.36). The remaining demographic features were similar between groups and are shown in Table 1.

Table 1. Demographic features between patients with major depression and anxiety disorders

	Depression (n = 70)		Anxiety (n = 88)		Statistics
	n	%	n	%	
Sex					
Men	12	17.1	27	30.7	$x^2 = 3.84$, df 1, p = 0.05
Women	58	82.9	61	69.3	
Marital status					
Single	35	50.0	45	51.1	$x^2 = 0.02$, df 1, p = 0.88
Married	35	50.0	43	48.9	
Laboral status					
Unemployed	50	71.4	54	61.4	$x^2 = 1.75$, df 1, p = 0.18
Employed	20	28.6	34	38.6	
Socioeconomic status					
Low	32	45.7	37	42.0	$x^2 = 3.93$, df 2, p = 0.14
Medium	20	28.6	37	42.0	
High	18	25.7	14	15.9	
	Mean	SD	Mean	SD	
Age	56.1	15.3	50.4	15.7	t = 2.28, df 156, p = 0.02
Length of education (years)	9.70	4.5	10.4	4.4	t = -1.09, df 156, p = 0.27

BZDs Use Features

Mean age of first BZD prescription was at 42.8 years (S.D. = 16.6, range 13-78 years), with an average time of consumption of 411.2 weeks (S.D. = 539, range 2-3250 weeks) equivalent to almost 8 years of consumption. The presence of anxious symptoms was the most frequent reason for BZD prescription (67.7%, n = 107) followed by insomnia (32.3%, n = 51). According to the SCID-I interview for dependence, 50.6% (n = 80) of the included patients report BZD dependence, with a moderate/severe pattern of severity (58.8%, n = 47 from those who exhibit BZD dependence). The mean scores of the BDEPQ-MX for the total sample were mild/moderate with a total score of 24.5 (S.D. = 17.3). However, these scores were significantly higher in those patients reporting BZD dependence: perceived need subscale mean score (13.4 vs. 5.1, $p < 0.001$), pleasant effects subscale mean score (9.4 vs. 4.1, $p < 0.001$), general dependence subscale mean score (12.5 vs 3.9, $p < 0.001$) and BDEPQ-MX total score (35.4 vs. 13.2, $p < 0.001$).

The comparison of BZD use features between patients with depression and anxiety disorders are displayed in Table 2. As can be seen, patients with anxiety disorders has an earlier age of onset of BZDs use (Cohen's d = 0.41), but total duration of BZD use was similar in both groups. Although anxiety was the primary reason for BZD prescription in both groups (52.9% for depressive patients and 79.5% for anxious patients), prescription due to insomnia was more frequent in patient with depression (47.1% vs. 20.5%, $p < 0.001$, Cramer's V = 0.28). For BZD dependence, a higher proportion of patients with anxiety were positive according to the SCID-I interview (58.0% vs. 41.4%, $p = 0.03$, Cramer's V = 0.16), although moderate/severe intensity of dependence was similar in both groups as well as the BDEPQ-MX scores. As prescription due to insomnia was more frequent in patients with depression, we decided to compare the BDEPQ-MX scores between depressive patients in accordance to the reason for BZD description (anxiety vs. insomnia). BDEPQ-MX scores were similar between groups except for the dimension "perceived need" where depressive patients under BZD due to anxious symptoms reported higher "perceived need" than those where BZD prescription was due to insomnia (10.7, S.D. = 7.7 vs. 6.7, S.D. = 6.6, t = 2.3, $p = 0.02$, Cohen d = 0.55).

Table 2. BZD use features between patients with major depression and anxiety disorders

	Depression (n = 70)		Anxiety (n = 88)		Statistics
	n	%	n	%	
Reason for prescription					
Anxious symptoms	37	52.9	70	79.5	$x^2 = 12.70$, df 1, $p < 0.001$
Insomnia	33	47.1	18	20.5	
BZD Dependence					
No	41	58.6	37	42.0	$x^2 = 4.26$, df 1, $p = 0.03$
Yes	29	41.4	51	58.0	
BZD Dependence Severity					
Mild	9	31.0	24	47.1	$x^2 = 1.95$, df 1, $p = 0.16$
Moderate/Severe	20	69.0	27	52.9	
	Mean	SD	Mean	SD	
Age of 1st BZD prescription	46.6	17.9	39.7	14.90	$t = 2.63$, df 156, $p = 0.009$
Time of consumption-weeks	388.7	528.6	429.1	550.0	$t = -0.46$, df 156, $p = 0.64$
BDEPQ-MX					
General dependence	8.4	8.1	8.1	6.7	$t = 0.24$, df 156, $p = 0.80$
Pleasant effects	7.0	5.0	6.6	4.5	$t = 0.41$, df 156, $p = 0.67$
Perceived need	8.8	7.4	9.7	6.6	$t = -0.81$, df 156, $p = 0.41$
Total score	24.3	19.4	24.6	15.6	$t = -0.11$, df 156, $p = 0.91$

The logistic regression models were significant for both groups according to the Hosmer & Lemeshaw statistical value (p > 0.05). The results of the logistic regression models showed that time of consumption was a risk factor for BZD dependence in both groups (anxiety, OR = 1.005; depression OR = 1.01), while being a male (OR = 0.29) was a protective factor for dependence in patients with anxiety disorders and being younger for patients with depression (OR = 0.72) (Table 3).

Table 3. Risk factors for BZD dependence in patients with major depression and anxiety disorders

	Depression			Anxiety		
	β	OR (C.I.)	p	β	OR (C.I.)	p
Initial Model						
Age	-0.33	0.71 (0.51-0.99)	0.04	0.04	1.04 (0.93-1.17)	0.41
Sex	1.00	2.74 (0.32-23.17)	0.35	-1.59	0.20 (0.05-0.81)	0.02
Marital – single	-1.11	0.33 (0.07-1.41)	0.13	-0.05	0.95 (0.31-2.88)	0.92
Employed	0.66	1.93 (0.30-12.24)	0.48	-0.30	0.74 (0.17-3.16)	0.68
Years of education	0.06	1.06 (0.88-1.27)	0.52	-0.01	0.98 (0.84-1.15)	0.88
Socioeconomic status	-0.28	0.74 (0.29-1.88)	0.54	0.37	1.45 (0.65-3.25)	0.36
Age of first BZD use	0.31	1.37 (1.01-1.85)	0.04	-0.03	0.96 (0.88-1.06)	0.51
Reason prescription	-0.53	0.58 (0.13-2.52)	0.47	0.48	1.62 (0.41-6.34)	0.48
Time of consumption	0.01	1.01 (1.005-1.02)	0.002	0.004	1.004 (1.000-1.008)	0.03
Final Model						
Age	-0.32	0.72 (0.52-0.99)	0.04	--	--	--
Sex	--	--	--	-1.23	0.29 (0.09-0.90)	0.03
Marital – single	-1.37	0.25 (0.06-1.02)	0.054	--	--	--
Age of 1st BZD use	0.29	1.34 (0.99-1.81)	0.057	--	--	--
Time of consumption	0.01	1.01 (1.004-1.01)	0.003	0.005	1.005 (1.002-1.009)	0.001

DISCUSSION

The objective of the present study was to compare BZD use between patients with major depression and anxiety disorders to determine which demographic features are related to BZD use and risk factors for BZD dependence. Our findings confirmed the high prevalence of BZD dependence amongst patients with anxiety and depressive disorders, where half of the patients fulfilled criteria for dependence (O'brien 2005; Minaya et al. 2011; Minaya, Ugalde, and Fresán 2009). Time of prescription also proved to be the main risk factor for developing BZD dependence (Menif et al. 2019). However, the main finding is that the characteristics of the population which develop dependence to these substances differs from one group to the other: while one should be especially careful when prescribing women with BZD for anxiety disorders regardless of age, it is older patients that are the most vulnerable to BZD dependence, regardless of gender, in depressive disorders.

Another interesting finding is that the reason for prescription differs between these populations: although anxiety was the main reason for prescription in both groups, insomnia seems to be relevant only in the depressed group. Also, depressed patients who take BZD for anxiety have a significantly higher perceived-need than those whose primary prescription is for insomnia. This could be explained from different perspectives. Our first hypothesis is that this difference could reside in the fact that patients with major depression, as mentioned by Barbui et al. (2011) are more likely to be treated in parallel with antidepressants than patients with anxious disorders. Antidepressants are frequently used off-label for the treatment of insomnia (Everitt et al. 2018) as some of them have sedative effects and guidelines for treatment of depressive disorders recommend choosing the antidepressant based on its side-effects profile (Lam et al. 2009; Stahl and Stahl 2013). Given the sedative effect, relief of insomnia is immediate and might even be equivalent to the relief provided by BZD, although we could not find evidence on the subject; as stated by Everitt et al. (2018) in their Cochrane review, there is little research on antidepressants and insomnia despite its frequent use in clinical settings. On the other hand, immediate relief of anxious symptoms is definitely not provided by antidepressants (which take from 4 to 6 weeks to provide relief in these symptoms) (Wichniak, Wierzbicka, and Jernajczyk 2012), making the perceived-need in this segment of the population much higher.

Model 1. Scenarios of treatment to cope with stressful situations

Scenario 1. Treatment: Benzodiazepines in monotherapy

Evolution in time	Exposure	Emotional reaction	Immediate treatment for this reaction	Emotion after treatment
t0	Difficult situation	Anxiety ++++	BZD standard dose	Anxiety +
t1	Same difficult situation	Anxiety ++++	BZD slightly higher dose	Anxiety +
t2	Same difficult situation	Anxiety ++++	BZD slightly higher dose	Anxiety +
tn	Same difficult situation	Anxiety ++++	BZD slightly higher dose	Anxiety +

Scenario 2. Treatment: Antidepressants and/or psychotherapy

Evolution in time	Exposure	Emotional reaction	Immediate treatment for this reaction	Emotion after treatment
t0	Difficult situation	Anxiety ++++	BZD standard dose	Anxiety ++
t1	Same difficult situation	Anxiety +++	BZD lower dose	Anxiety +
t2	Same difficult situation	Anxiety +	No BZD required	--
tn	Same difficult situation	Discomfort	No BZD required	--

In scenario Num. 1 BZD are the only treatment. Therefore, treatment is mainly focused on alleviating the unpleasant immediate emotion triggered by a difficult (stressful) situation. The emotional response to the stressful situation remains unchanged, and there is a need for increasing doses of BZD to achieve the same response (tolerance).

In scenario Num. 2, although BZD are part of the treatment with an intention to lower the intensity of the unpleasant immediate emotion, the goal is achieving a better control of emotional responses. Therefore, as treatment evolves, the emotional response improves until stressful situations become manageable without palliatives.

t0, t1, t3, tn: Time 0 (first exposure), time 1 (second exposure), time 2 (third exposure), time n (any number of subsequent exposures).

Another hypothesis (proposed model 1), concordant with the previous, is that the long-term use of benzodiazepines in monotherapy for anxious symptoms delays the adaptation of the subject to stressful situations. Some degree of discomfort might help the subject search for efficacious coping strategies (Charney 2003), however BZD in high doses could eradicate discomfort, making the search for different strategies unnecessary.

This study outlined important differences in the risk factors associated to BZD dependence in major depressive disorder and anxiety disorders. It has however, some limitations: the cross-sectional design impedes analyses of possible changes in severity of usage over time. Also, other factors such as personality disorders, concomitant treatment with other drugs and non-pharmacological treatments were not accounted for and could influence our results.

In conclusion, we believe further studies assessing safety and effectiveness of other alternative medications for symptoms where BZDs are prescribed are necessary to develop complementary treatments without the clinical risks associated to BZDs use. Moreover, clinicians and patients should be encouraged to consider and trained to use alternative medications to BZD, such as antidepressants, antipsychotic drugs, alternative hypnotics, as well as non-pharmacological interventions that have already proven to be safer and very effective to manage a variety of conditions that by uses and custom are treated with BDZ, such as anxiety and insomnia. For example, the cognitive-behavioral therapy for insomnia (CBT-I) (van Straten, et al., 2018), a structured intervention that typically incorporates education about the behaviors and routines that promote sleep, behavioral techniques like stimulus control, and training on relaxation, deep diaphragmatic breathing or mindfulness, as well as cognitive components including the identification and modification of worries and thoughts that prevent the person from falling asleep, and paradoxical intention (Luik, et al., 2019), which is considered by the American and European guidelines as the first-line treatment for insomnia disorder (Qaseem, Kansagara, Forciea, Cooke, and Denberg, 2016; Riemann et al., 2017).

Given that the implementation of this kind of non-pharmacological interventions requires more effort from both the clinician and the patient in comparison with pill intake, it is essential to inform about the benefit that would be obtained through this additional work to avoid the long-term use and BZD dependence.

Finally, clinicians should bear in mind socio-demographic characteristics of vulnerable population. Although the effectivity of BZDs has been proven, clinicians alongside patients need to establish clear and specific goals regarding the use of BZD.

REFERENCES

Airagnes, G., Lemogne, C., Renuy, A., Goldberg, M., Hoertel, N., Roquelaure, Y., … Zins, M. (2019). Prevalence of prescribed benzodiazepine long-term use in the French general population according to sociodemographic and clinical factors: findings from the CONSTANCES cohort. *BMC Public Health,* 19(1), 566. https://doi.org/10.1186/s12889-019-6933-8.

Baillie, A., & Mattick, R. (1996). The Benzodiazepine Dependence Questionnaire: development, reliability and validity. *Br. J. Psychiatry,* 169, 276−281. https://doi.org/10.1192/bjp.169.3.276.

Bandelow, B., Zohar, J., Hollander, E., Kasper, S., & Möller, H.J. (2008). World Federation of Societies of Biological Psychiatry (WFSBP) guidelines for the pharmacological treatment of anxiety, obsessive-compulsive and post-traumatic stress disorders--first revision. *World J. Biol. Psychiatry,* 9(4), 248–312. https://doi.org/10.1080/15622970802465807.

Barbui, C., Cipriani, A., Patel, V., Ayuso-Mateos, J. L., & van Ommeren, M. (2011). Efficacy of antidepressants and benzodiazepines in minor depression: systematic review and meta-analysis. *Br. J. Psychiatry,* 198(1), 11–16, suppl 1. https://doi.org/10.1192/bjp.bp.109.076448.

Bushnell, G. A., Stürmer, T., Gaynes, B. N., Pate, V., & Miller, M. (2017). Simultaneous antidepressant and benzodiazepine new Use and Subsequent Long-term Benzodiazepine Use in Adults with Depression, United States, 2001-2014. *JAMA Psychiatry,* 74(7), 747–755. https://doi.org/10.1001/jamapsychiatry.2017.1273.

Charney, D. S. (2003). The psychobiology of resilience and vulnerability to anxiety disorders: implications for prevention and treatment. *Dialogues Clin. Neurosci,* 5(3), 207–221. PMC3181630.

Ciuna, A., Andretta, M., Corbari, L., Levi, D., Mirandola, M., Sorio, A., & Barbui, C. (2004). Are we going to increase the use of antidepressants up to that of benzodiazepines? *Eur. J. Clin. Pharmacol,* 60(9), 629–634. https://doi.org/10.1007/s00228-004-0810-8.

Crowe, S. F., & Stranks, E. K. (2018). The Residual Medium and Long-term Cognitive Effects of Benzodiazepine Use: An Updated Meta-analysis. *Arch. Clin. Neuropsychol,* 33(7), 901–911. https://doi.org/10.1093/arclin/acx120.

Everitt, H., Baldwin, D. S., Stuart, B., Lipinska, G., Mayers, A., Malizia, A. L., … Wilson, S. (2018). Antidepressants for insomnia in adults. *Cochrane Database Syst. Rev.,* 5, CD010753. https://doi.org/10.1002/14651858.CD010753.pub2.

Fang, S. Y., Chen, C. Y., Chang, I. S., Wu, E. C. H., Chang, C. M., & Lin, K. M. (2009). *Predictors of the incidence and discontinuation of long-term use of benzodiazepines: A population-based study.* Drug Alcohol Depend, 104(1-2), 140–146. https://doi.org/10.1016/j.drugalcdep.2009.04.017.

Fassaert, T., Dorn, T., Spreeuwenberg, P. M. M., van Dongen, M. C. J. M., van Gool, C. J. A. W., & Yzermans, C. J. (2007). Prescription of benzodiazepines in general practice in the context of a man-made disaster: a longitudinal study. *Eur. J. Public Health,* 17(6), 612–617. https://doi.org/10.1093/eurpub/ckm020.

First M, Spitzer R, Gibbon M, Williams J (1996). *Structured Clinical Interview for DSM-IV Axis I Disorders (SCID-I),* Clinician Version. Washington, D.C.: American Psychiatric Press.

Greenblatt, D. J., Harmatz, J. S., & Shader, R. I. (2018). Update on Psychotropic Drug Prescribing in the United States: 2014–2015. *J. Clin. Psychopharmacol.,* 38(1), 1. https://doi.org/10.1097/JCP.0000000000000831

Howard, P., Twycross, R., Shuster, J., Mihaylo, M., & Wilcock, A. (2014). Benzodiazepines. *Journal of Pain and Symptom Management, 47*(5), 955–964. https://doi.org/10.1016/j.jpainsymman.2014.03.001.

Kanazawa, T., Hamada, T., Nishihara, M., Ian, A., Yoneda, H., Nakajima, M., & Katsumata, T. (2018). What can predict and prevent the long-term use of benzodiazepines? *J. Psychiatr. Res., 97,* 94–100. https://doi.org/10.1016/j.jpsychires.2017.11.012.

Lam, R. W., Kennedy, S. H., Grigoriadis, S., McIntyre, R. S., Milev, R., Ramasubbu, R., ... Ravindran, A. V. (2009). Canadian Network for Mood and Anxiety Treatments (CANMAT) clinical guidelines for the management of major depressive disorder in adults. III. Pharmacotherapy. *J. Affect. Disord.,* 117 Suppl, S26–S43. https://doi.org/10.1016/j.jad.2009.06.041.

Luik, A. I., van der Zweerde, T., van Straten, A., & Lancee, J. (2019). Digital Delivery of Cognitive Behavioral Therapy for Insomnia. *Curr. Psychiatry Rep., 21*(7), 50. https://doi.org/10.1007/s11920-019-1041-0.

Menif, L., Oueslati, B., Maamri, A., Melki, W., & Zalila, H. (2019). Correlates of benzodiazepine dependence in patients with depression followed up in a psychiatric outpatient unit in Tunisia. *J. Ethn. Subst. Abuse.,* 1–13. https://doi.org/10.1080/15332640.2019.1589611.

Minaya, O., Fresán, A., Cortes-Lopez, J. L., Nanni, R., & Ugalde, O. (2011). The Benzodiazepine Dependence Questionnaire (BDEPQ): validity and reliability in Mexican psychiatric patients. *Addict. Behav., 36*(8), 874–877. https://doi.org/10.1016/j.addbeh.2011.03.007.

Minaya, O., Ugalde, O., & Fresán, A. (2009). Uso inapropiado de fármacos de prescripción: dependencia a benzodiazepinas en adultos mayores [Prescription drug misuse: benzodiazepine dependence in the elderly]. *Salud Ment.* https://www.scielo.org.mx/pdf/sm/v32n5/v32n5a7.pdf.

Moylan, S., Staples, J., Ward, S. A., Rogerson, J., Stein, D. J., & Berk, M. (2011). The efficacy and safety of alprazolam versus other benzodiazepines in the treatment of panic disorder. *J. Clin. Psychopharmacol., 31*(5), 647–652. https://doi.org/10.1097/JCP.0b013e31822d0012.

O'brien, C. P. (2005). Benzodiazepine use, abuse, and dependence. *J. Clin. Psychiatry,* 66 Suppl 2, 28–33. https://www.ncbi.nlm.nih.gov/pubmed/15762817.

Ogawa, Y., Takeshima, N., Hayasaka, Y., Tajika, A., Watanabe, N., Streiner, D., & Furukawa, T. A. (2019). Antidepressants plus benzodiazepines for adults with major depression. *Cochrane Database Syst. Rev.,* 6, CD001026. https://doi.org/10.1002/14651858.CD001026.pub2.

Qaseem, A., Kansagara, D., Forciea, M. A., Cooke, M., & Denberg, T. D. (2016). Management of Chronic Insomnia Disorder in Adults: A Clinical Practice Guideline from the American College of Physicians. *Ann of Intern Med,* 165(2), 125–133. https://doi.org/10.7326/m15-2175.

Richardson, M., O'Dwyer, C., Gaskin, J., Conyard, E., & Murphy, K. D. (2019). A study to evaluate the potential contribution of medication use to falls in elderly patients presenting to an acute hospital. *Hospital Pharmacists Association of Ireland Annual Conference* 2019. https://cora.ucc.ie/handle/10468/7831.

Riemann, D., Baglioni, C., Bassetti, C., Bjorvatn, B., Groselj, L. D., Ellis, J. G., ... Spiegelhalder, K. (2017). European guideline for the diagnosis and treatment of insomnia. *J Sleep Res,* 26(6), 675–700. https://doi.org/10.1111/jsr.12594.

Sjöstedt, C., Ohlsson, H., Li, X., & Sundquist, K. (2017). Sociodemographic factors and long-term use of benzodiazepines in patients with depression, anxiety or insomnia. *Psychiatry Res.,* 249, 221–225. https://doi.org/10.1016/j.psychres.2017.01.046.

Stahl, S. M., & Stahl, S. M. (2013). *Stahl's Essential Psychopharmacology: Neuroscientific Basis and Practical Applications.* Cambridge University Press. United Kingdom. ISBN: 978-1-107-68646-5. https://www.cambridge.org/9781107025981.

van Straten, A., van der Zweerde, T., Kleiboer, A., Cuijpers, P., Morin, C. M., & Lancee, J. (2018). Cognitive and behavioral therapies in the treatment of insomnia: A meta-analysis. *Sleep Med. Rev.,* 38, 3–16. https://doi.org/10.1016/j.smrv.2017.02.001.

Villatoro, J., Medina-Mora, M., Fleiz Bautista, C., Moreno López, M., Oliva Robles, N., Bustos Gamiño, M., ... Amador Buenabad, N. (2012). El consumo de drogas en México: Resultados de la Encuesta Nacional de Adicciones, 2011 [Drug use in Mexico: Results from the 2011 National Addictions Survey]. *Salud Ment.,* 35(6), 447–457. http://www.scielo.org.mx/pdf/sm/v35n6/v35n6a1.pdf.

Wichniak, A., Wierzbicka, A., & Jernajczyk, W. (2012). Sleep and antidepressant treatment. *Curr. Pharm. Des.,* 18(36), 5802–5817. https://doi.org.10.2174/138161212803523608.

In: Depression and Anxiety
Editor: Shelley L. Becker

ISBN: 978-1-53617-229-4
© 2020 Nova Science Publishers, Inc.

Chapter 4

IMMUNOLOGY OF ANXIETY DISORDERS

Suprakash Chaudhury[1,]*, Satyam Kishore[2], Ajay K. Bakhla[3] and Swalwha Mujawar[1]

[1]Department of Psychiatry, Dr. D. Y. Patil Medical College, Dr. D. Y. Patil University, Pune, Maharshtra, India
[2]Department of Psychiatry, CIP, Ranchi, Jhankhand, India
[3]Department of Psychiatry, RIMS, Ranchi, Jhankhand, India

ABSTRACT

There has been increasing focus placed on immune mediated theories in understanding the underlying mechanisms of disorders like anxiety, posttraumatic stress, and obsessive compulsive disorders as the prevalence of these disorders continues to rise all over the world. Literature suggests correlations between the abnormalities in the hypothalamic–pituitary–adrenal (HPA) axis and these disorders, especially in terms of cortisol levels. This chapter systematically assesses the available research data in the last 10 years which sheds light on association between psychoneuroimmunology and anxiety. Finding out the underlying processes leading to these illnesses is crucial for specific

---

* Corresponding Author's Email: suprakashch@gmail.com.

and effective treatment strategies, giving rise to considerable improvement in overall functioning, and also considerable decreases in burden on the economy and society.

Keywords: anxiety disorders, HPA axis, cortisol, cytokines

INTRODUCTION

Earlier versions of the Diagnostic and Statistical Manual of Mental Disorders (DSM) up to DSM IV TR included the following under anxiety disorders: generalized anxiety disorder, panic disorder, post-traumatic stress disorder, social anxiety disorder, specific phobia and obsessive compulsive disorder. However, the latest version of DSM (DSM 5) now classifies PTSD under Trauma- and Stressor-Related Disorders and OCD under Obsessive-Compulsive and Related Disorders [1]. The lifetime prevalence rate of these disorders was found to be as high as 28.3% worldwide [2] which results in high economic costs especially the extensive utilization of primary care services. Hence, further understanding of the causes of these disorders may lead to decrease in the treatment costs and improvement in the patient outcome. This recently increased interest has been placed on psychoneuroimmunology research, specifically in regard to anxiety disorders, PTSD and OCD. There is an increased risk of comorbid neurological, vascular, respiratory, and metabolic conditions in such patients.

A lot of studies have been done regarding the relationship between stress and immune function, but most of these reports deal with the acute effects of experimental or artificial stress. Others have studied the association between immune or endocrine functions with chronic or predictable stressful situations like death of spouse, caring for the disabled, upcoming examinations, etc.

It has been commonly seen that many factors such as stress and depression have been shown to influence the immune system in terms of immunosuppression and immune activation [3]. Anxiety disorders show activation of the immune system and differentiation or death of certain cells and changes in levels of certain chemokines and growth factors like brain-derived neurotrophic factor, interleukins (ILs), tumour necrosis factors (TNFs), interferons (IFNs), etc. [4]. Hence, there is a complex interaction between reactions to stress by the HPA axis, immune function and changes in mood.

Dearth of information about the long-term effects of acute stress is predominantly important. It has been observed that within 3 months of mourning, a study group comprising of widows had lesser CD19qCD5q B cell subpopulation.

They were also found to have greater proliferation responses to PHA, anti-CD3 and PWM. There was no significant difference found between widows and non-widows in NK cell concentration. The same subjects showed no significant differences in the total number of white blood cells, number of lymphocyte subsets and NK cell concentration after seven months of bereavement.

Despite these findings, physical illness and mortality were found to be increased during the first two years of bereavement, and this vulnerability could be attributable to the persistent activation of the adrenocortical axis and altered immune function following bereavement, with long-lasting brain changes involving neurotransmitters, neuropeptides and receptors [5].

In asymptomatic HIV type 1-seropositive homosexual men, bereavement was found to be associated with time-dependent decrements in cellular immune function [6], and immune decrements were associated with increased neuroendocrine responses of the sympathetic adrenomedullary system as well as the limbic-hypothalamic-pituitary-adrenal axis.

However, the exact relationships between psychological status and long-term immune responses to stress with the probable variability related to personality factors and mood are still not properly understood. The present chapter will comprehensively review scientific literature from the past decade, specifically related to psychoneuroimmunology in anxiety, posttraumatic stress, and obsessive compulsive disorders.

PSYCHOIMMUNOLOGY AND CYTOKINES

Since the establishment of links between pro- and anti-inflammatory biomarkers, there has been a rise in use of molecular and immunological research techniques in evaluating people with psychiatric illnesses. The HPA axis is activated during stressful events which leads to secretion of corticotropin releasing hormone (CRH) and arginine vasopressin (AVP) leading to the release of adrenocorticotropic hormone (ACTH) which stimulates the release of cortisol and glucocorticoids. The interaction between the central nervous system (CNS) and peripheral immune system is carried out by cytokines like tumor necrosis factor-alpha (TNF-α) and interleukins (IL) 2 and 6. Moreover, they also lead to the formation of other cytokines. These cytokines initiate immune processes like allergic response, are involved in repair mechanisms after any injury, and control the endocrine system via HPA axis [7].

T-helper cells are of two types based on the kind of cytokines produced by them. They are the Th1 cells which secrete cytokines IL-2, TNF-α and interferon-γ (IFN-γ) and the Th2 cells which secrete cytokines IL-4, 5, 6, 10, 13. They play a role in activating cell-mediated and humoral immunity [8]. An imbalance between Th1 and Th2 cytokines is seen in psychiatric illnesses like anxiety, PTSD, and OCD etc. These illnesses are often accompanied by a shift from a Th1/Th2 balance to Th2 dominance. There is increase in IL-6 and TNF-α [9]. Additionally, decreased Th1 cytokines and a shift towards Th2 leads to deficits in serotonergic activity giving rise to symptoms of anxiety [10].

A very important factor affecting the inflammatory response is the balance between Th1 and Th2 [11]. Research shows that T helper type 3 cells secrete transforming growth factor beta-1 which is known to maintain the balance between the Th1 and Th2 [12]. A normal neuropsychiatric functioning needs equilibrium between the pro–inflammatory and anti-inflammatory cytokines [13]. The neuronal functions in areas like the cerebral cortex, hippocampus, amygdala and hypothalamus are affected by certain cytokines [14, 15]. The cytokine expression in the brain is affected by factors such as presence of infection, inflammation or stress [16].

The ways by which these chemicals reach the CNS are as follows:

1. Passing via a "leaky" area in the blood–brain barrier.
2. Brain endothelium containing specific transport systems.
3. The release of second messengers after stimulation of endothelial cells.
4. Vagus nerve which carries the afferent signals.
5. Stimulated monocyte cells cause entry of these chemicals in the CNS [17].

The cytokines exert their action through the following mechanisms:

1. Causing changes in the metabolism of dopamine, serotonin and glutamate [18-20].
2. Causing changes in the HPA axis and subsequently leading to release of cortisol [21, 22].
3. Causing activation of nuclear factor kappa-light-chain-enhancer of B cells leading to neurogenesis [23].
4. Affecting the anterior cingulate cortex (dorsal part), and basal ganglia areas of the brain [24, 25].

PSYCHONEUROIMMUNOLOGY IN ANXIETY DISORDERS

One of the main causes of anxiety is the activation of HPA axis by chronic stress [26]. It was seen that autoimmune mice with anxiety had greater levels of cytokines in animal studies [27-29].

Certain medical conditions like diabetes, cardiovascular disorders, and autoimmune diseases like rheumatoid arthritis are associated with anxiety disorders. It is expected that the disability is more when anxiety disorders are accompanied by medical conditions when compared with a state when the medical condition is existing alone. Compared to healthy individuals the subjects with rheumatoid arthritis (RA) have a higher levels of IL-17, TNF-α, and IL-6. However, patients with both RA and anxiety show higher IL-17 and these levels positively and independently correlate with the severity of anxiety [30]. A study found correlation between anxiety and IFN- levels in patients with systemic lupus erythematous [31].

Impaired immunological reaction to many vaccines like pneumococcal bacteria [32], hepatitis B virus [33], rubella virus [34], meningitis virus [35] and influenza virus [36-38] is also seen in anxiety.

There is increasing focus on evaluating the association between the immune system and psychiatric disorders to recognise further the mechanisms giving rise to these disorders. This research is required for better medications specifically targeted at these biomarkers in study populations ranging from children, adolescents, adults, to the elderly. We will now consider these in different anxiety disorders.

Generalized Anxiety Disorder

Generalized Anxiety Disorder (GAD) is found in around 1.9 – 5.1% of the people in the general population and around 8% of individuals coming to primary care [39]. This disorder is characterized by excessive worrying thoughts which have lasted for at least six months duration and are usually regarding daily activities like relationships, health, work and finances [1].

A T cell dysfunction was seen in patients with GAD by studying the T cells after in vitro activation in cultures. It was also found that in GAD, Th1 and Th2 deficiencies were associated with dominant Th17 phenotype, which was increased by substance P [40, 41].

Changes in C - reactive protein (CRP) levels are found in subjects diagnosed with GAD. A significantly increased cortisol is seen more in GAD especially in female children and adolescents. Additionally, these raised cortisol levels anticipated greater symptom severity at the 12-month follow-up for females. A strong correlation between CRP and GAD was found in stable coronary heart disease patients [42]. A research was done comparing the levels of the proinflammatory cytokines monocyte chemoattractant protein-1 (MCP-1), chemokine C-C motif ligand 5 (CCL-5) and stromal derived factor-1 (SDF-1) in GAD patients having comorbid personality disorder with healthy controls. It was found that levels of MCP-1 and SDF-1 in both the sexes were more, and elevated CCL-5 was found in men but not women with a diagnosis of GAD when compared to the control group [43].

The evaluation of variation in HPA activity has been used to assess the efficacy of pharmacological treatment in anxiety. A randomized, double-blind, placebo-controlled trial including GAD patients was undertaken to find out how SSRI treatment affects HPA activity. A higher cortisol levels and higher reduction in both peak and total cortisol levels after escitalopram treatment was found in GAD patients when compared to placebo [44].

Changes in cortisol levels and corrections in symptom severity are seen after psychotherapy. The efficacy of cognitive therapy (CT) in association with cortisol levels was evaluated in GAD patients. Hair cortisol levels (3 hair segments) were assessed in patients diagnosed with GAD compared to matched controls. The investigators undertook a total of 12 saliva collections (awakening, 30min, 12:00, 16:00, 20:00, and bedtime) on consecutive weekdays. When compared to controls, the cortisol levels in the hair were found to be lower in GAD patients. The cortisol levels in saliva were found to be similar in both groups. However, research done in the past showed higher cortisol in saliva and plasma in subjects with anxiety [45, 46].

Social Anxiety Disorder

Social Anxiety Disorder (SAD) may develop as early as 11years of age in almost 50% of the cases [47]. It consequently becomes important to evaluate all possible processes causing this disorder like prenatal risk factors.

Due to this early age-of-onset, patients with anxiety predictably undergo substantial problems in social skills development giving rise to problems in coping skills which are important in socialization during childhood, adolescence and adulthood.

Higher bedtime cortisol levels from baseline to first week of school were seen in children of socially anxious mothers, apart from raised cortisol levels in the morning and afternoon. Conversely, children without socially anxious mothers only displayed rise in cortisol levels in morning and afternoon. These results were the first to establish variation in HPA activity in children who are at a greater risk of developing SAD [48].

Panic Disorder

According to the American Psychiatric Association having unexpected panic attacks and the continuous fear of experiencing these attacks again along with a change in behaviour to avoid these attacks which is present for a minimum duration of one month leads to a diagnosis of Panic Disorder (PD) [1]. HPA axis activity in symptomatic people with PD, asymptomatic PD people who were treated and healthy controls were exposed to a simulated public speaking (SPS) exercise while salivary cortisol levels were measured.

The Visual Analog Mood Scale (VAMS), State-Trait Anxiety Inventory-Trait form (STAI-T), and the Bodily Symptoms Scale (BSS) were used to evaluate the severity of anxiety. As would be predicted, scores on the VAMS and BSS were increased in symptomatic patients compared to the asymptomatic patients. It was found that cortisol levels did not rise due to the SPS, showing that public speaking may not particularly cause activation of HPA. Possibly, HPA over-activation may be theorised exclusively to individuals suffering from fear of public speaking [49]. Nonetheless, in patients with PD, HPA over activity may be linked with panic attacks [50].

Abnormal levels of IL-1 have been reported in patients with PD [51]. The effectiveness of medicines in changing immune activity was studied in subjects with PD, either alone or in combination with CBT to find if there are any variations in phytohemagglutinin (PHA) and IL-2 levels [52]. HAM-A scores, Korean version of the Symptom Checklist-90 Revised (SCL-90-R) anxiety subscale scores, PHA-induced production, IL-2 production were found to be higher in patients before treatment as compared to controls.

There is a need for more research studying long term effects of various possible treatment options. A direct association between HPA activity and SAD resulting in heightened levels of cortisol has been shown after stress and avoidance behaviour [53]. Moreover, compared to blood pressure and subjective anxiety, cortisol levels had a higher predictive effect on avoidance, proving the role of the HPA axis in adult patients with SAD.

Posttraumatic Stress Disorder

According to the DSM 5 Posttraumatic Stress Disorder (PTSD) is no longer part of anxiety disorder, but is now reclassified under "Trauma- and Stressor-Related Disorder" [1].

Kawamura et al. reported that there is suppression of the cellular immunity in men with a history of post-traumatic stress disorder (PTSD) in the past. They found that the number of lymphocytes and T cells, NK cell activity, and total amounts of interferon-gamma and interleukin 4 were considerably lesser in subjects with PTSD, showing long-lasting immunosuppression and therefore dire implications for their health. When compared to controls, the parents who had faced sudden demise of a previously healthy child were found to have lower T-suppressor cells, higher T-helper cells, and depression with no significant difference in cortisol levels [54]. Research suggests that cellular immunity is a factor in PTSD risk [55]. There are raised levels of TNF-a, CRP, IL-6, IL -1b and IL-8 in PTSD patients possibly because of abnormal regulation of immune function [56, 57].

HPA activity is abnormal in persons with PTSD. This results in abnormal levels of cortisol, due to a change in Th1/Th2 balance to Th2 dominance [58].

The emphasis of immunology research in psychiatric disorders is shifting towards the abnormal regulation in proinflammatory cytokines that hypothetically leads to increase in inflammation. A study was carried out on 2555 marines and sailors to evaluate PTSD after deployment. Baseline CRP plasma concentration was found to be a good predictor of PTSD symptoms [59].

We could use this to possibly suggest sites where treatments could be developed to target abnormal inflammatory levels, and decrease symptom severity in PTSD patients. Nevertheless, more studies are needed to corroborate this hypothesis.

Increased levels of CRP and IL-6 were found in Police officers suffering from PTSD [60]. A decreased salivary cortisol and increased DHEA, TNF-α, and IL-6 was seen in females with PTSD when compared to females without PTSD [61]. Furthermore, comorbid MDD was associated with higher abnormalities in the HPA axis. Additionally, the frequency of interpersonal violence was found to escalate the CRP levels [61]. Individuals subjected to the 9/11 attacks were interviewed and evaluated for PTSD symptoms by the self-report Perceived Stress Scale (PSS). Baseline cortisol levels predicted cortisol levels after the interview. Interestingly, in male subjects, higher cortisol levels indicated higher severity of re-experiencing PTSD symptoms that may imply a sex-specific mechanism of HPA abnormality [62].

Obsessive Compulsive Disorder

Even though obsessive–compulsive disorder (OCD) is commonly seen in psychiatric setups, its causal processes are not fully understood. Paediatric Autoimmune Neuropsychiatric Disorders Associated with Streptococcal infections (PANDAS) which is a subtype of OCD is thought to originate via immune mediated processes. A lot of research involving early-onset OCD has been dedicated to establish an association between newly acquired group A beta hemolytic streptococcal infections and symptom exacerbations, finding antineural antibodies which might cause the illness, and the occurrence of the D8/17 surface antigen on lymphocytes. However, no conclusive findings are there. A few researches have focussed on the potential role of cytokines and T cell function in these disorders especially in adults.

Studies have found a reduction in production of TNF-α and the low levels of lipopolysacacharide-stimulated IL-6 in OCD [63, 64]. However, a few others reported IL-6 differences in cerebrospinal fluid or in plasma [65, 66].

Another study found greater levels of TNF-α and IL-6 in OCD patients [67].

CONCLUSION

There have been recent studies on the interactions between the central nervous system, agents causing infection, and the immunological system especially the cytokines. Researchers have pointed to cytokines in the pathogenesis of a number of psychiatric illnesses like depression, schizophrenia, dementia, and post-traumatic stress disorder.

Patients with various forms of anxiety, obsessive compulsive disorder, and posttraumatic stress disorder suffer from a lot of stress leading to many changes which also include dysfunctions in the immune system. The dysfunctions of HPA axis and pro- and anti-inflammatory cytokines is especially seen in anxiety related illnesses.

Increased HPA activity is seen in the anxious subjects and a decrease in HPA activity after treatment with SSRIs and cognitive therapy. PTSD and OCD show increased cytokines like IL-6 and TNF-α. Since, earlier reports have proved that cortisol levels are indicative of PTSD diagnosed in soldiers after deployment and in new-borns with mothers suffering from obsessive compulsive disorder, studying the immune system and these specific biomarkers are crucial for recognizing how to deal with these disorders.

In order to decrease individual burden and also the burden on society in people suffering from anxiety and other related disorders we need to focus on markers for acute stress and chronic stress and also markers for specific disorders.

REFERENCES

[1] American Psychiatric Association, 2013. *Diagnostic and Statistical Manual of Mental Disorders*, 5th ed. American Psychiatric Publishing, Arlington.

[2] Baxter, A. J., Scott, K. M., Vos, T. and Whiteford, H. A. (2013). Global prevalence of anxiety disorders: a systematic review and meta-regression. *Psychological Medicine*, 43 (5), 897 - 910.

[3] Raison, C. L. and Miller, A. H. (2001). The neuroimmunology of stress and depression. *Seminars in Clinical Neuropsychiatry*, 6 (4), 277 - 294.

[4] Allan, S. M. and Rothwell, N. J. (2003). Inflammation in central nervous system injury. *Philos. Trans. R Soc. Lond. B Biol. Sci.*, 358, 1669 - 1677.

[5] Biondi, M. and Picardi, A. (1996). Clinical and biological aspects of bereavement and loss-induced depression: a reappraisal. *Psychotherapy and Psychosomatics*, 65, 229 - 245.

[6] Goodkin, K., Feaster, D. J., Tuttle, R., Blaney, N. T., Kumar, M., Baum, M. K., Shapshak, P. and Fletcher, M. A. (1996). Bereavement is associated with time-dependent decrements in cellular immune function in asymptomatic human immunodeficiency virus type 1-seropositive homosexual men. *Clinical and Diagnostic Laboratory Immunology,* 3, 109 - 118.

[7] Kasper, S., den Boer, J. A. and Sitsen, J. M. (2003). *Handbook of Depression and Anxiety: A Biological Approach*, 2nd Ed. Marcel Dekker Inc., New York.

[8] Glik, A. and Douvdevani, A. (2006). T lymphocytes: the "cellular" arm of acquired immunity in the peritoneum. *Perit. Dial. Int.*, 26(4), 438 - 48.

[9] Martino, D. J., Bosco, A., McKenna, K. L., Hollams, E., Mok, D., Holt, P. G. and Prescott, S. L. (2012). T-cell activation gene differentially expressed at birth in CD4+ T-cells from children who develop IgE food allergy. *Allergy,* 67, 191 - 200.

[10] Fernandez, S. P. and Gaspar, P. (2012). Investigating anxiety and depressive-like phenotypes in genetic mouse models of serotonin depletion. *Neuropharmacology,* 62(1), 144 - 154.

[11] Dantzer, R., Capuron, L., Irwin, M. R., Miller, A. H., Ollat, H., Perry, V. H., Rousey, S. and Yirmiya, R. (2008). Identification and treatment of symptoms associated with inflammation in medically ill patients. *Psychoneuroendocrinology,* 33, 18 - 29.

[12] Myint, A. M., Leonard, B. E., Steinbusch, H. W. and Kim, Y. K. (2005). Th1, Th2, and Th3 cytokine alterations in major depression. *J. Affect. Disord.,* 88, 167 - 173.

[13] Loftis, J. M., Huckans, M., Morasco, B. J. (2010). Neuroimmune mechanisms of cytokine-induced depression: current theories and novel treatment strategies. *Neurobiol. Dis.,* 37, 519 - 533.

[14] Besedovsky, H. O. and del Rey, A. (1996). Immune-neuro-endocrine interactions: facts and hypotheses. *Endocr. Rev.,* 17. 64 - 102.

[15] Elenkov, I. J., Wilder, R. L., Chrousos, G. P. and Vizi, E. S. (2000). The sympathetic nerve—an integrative interface between two supersystems: the brain and the immune system. *Pharmacol. Rev.,* 52, 595 - 638.

[16] Lucas, S. M., Rothwell, N. J. and Gibson, R. M. (2006). The role of inflammation in CNS injury and disease. *Br. J. Pharmacol.,* 147(Suppl. 1), S232 - S240.

[17] Capuron, L. and Miller, A. H. (2011). Immune system to brain signaling: neuropsychopharmacological implications. *Pharmacol. Ther.,* 130, 226 - 238.

[18] Moron, J. A., Zakharova, I., Ferrer J. V., Merrill, G. A., Hope, B., Lafer, E. M., Lin, Z. C., Wang, J. B., Javitch, J. A., Galli, A. and Shippenberg, T. S. (2003). Mitogen-activated protein kinase regulates dopamine transporter surface expression and dopamine transport capacity. *J. Neurosci.,* 23, 8480 - 8488.

[19] Cai, W., Khaoustov, V. I., Xie, Q., Pan, T., Le, W. and Yoffe, B. (2005). Interferonalpha-induced modulation of glucocorticoid and serotonin receptors as a mechanism of depression. *J. Hepatol.,* 42, 880 - 887.

[20] Ida, T., Hara, M., Nakamura, Y., Kozaki, S., Tsunoda, S. and Ihara, H. (2008). Cytokine-induced enhancement of calcium-dependent glutamate release from astrocytes mediated by nitric oxide. *Neurosci. Lett.,* 432, 232 - 236.

[21] Pariante, C. M. and Miller, A. H. (2001). Glucocorticoid receptors in major depression: relevance to pathophysiology and treatment. *Biol. Psychiatry,* 49, 391 - 404.

[22] Raison, C. L., Borisov, A. S., Woolwine, B. J., Massung, B., Vogt, G. and Miller, A. H. (2010). Interferon-alpha effects on diurnal hypothalamic–pituitary–adrenal axis activity: relationship with proinflammatory cytokines and behavior. *Mol. Psychiatry,* 15, 535 - 547.

[23] Menachem-Zidon, O. B., Goshen, I., Kreisel, T., Menahem, Y. B., Reinhartz, E., Hur, T. B. and Yirmiya, R. (2008). Intrahippocampal transplantation of transgenic neural precursor cells overexpressing interleukin-1 receptor antagonist blocks chronic isolation-induced impairment in memory and neurogenesis. *Neuropsychopharmacology,* 33, 2251 - 2262.

[24] Brydon, L., Harrison, N. A., Walker, C., Steptoe, A. and Critchley, H. D. (2008). Peripheral inflammation is associated with altered substantia nigra activity and psychomotor slowing in humans. *Biol. Psychiatry,* 63, 1022 - 1029.

[25] Miller, A. H. and Timmie, W. P. (2009). Mechanisms of Cytokine-Induced Behavioral Changes: Psychoneuroimmunology at the Translational Interface Norman Cousins Lecture. *Brain Behav. Immun.,* 23(2), 149 - 158.

[26] Leonard, B. E. and Myint, A. (2009). The psychoneuroimmunology of depression. *Hum. Psychopharmacol.,* 24, 165 - 175.

[27] Bluthe, R. M., Dantzer, R. and Kelley, K. W. (1992). Effects of interleukin-1 receptor antagonist on the behavioral effects of lipopolysaccharide in rat. *Brain Res.,* 573, 318 - 320.

[28] Sakic, B., Szechtman, H., Talangbayan, H., Denburg, S. D., Carbotte, R. M. and Denburg, J. A. (1994). Disturbed emotionality in autoimmune MRL-lpr mice. *Physiol. Behav.,* 56, 609 - 617.

[29] Schrott, L. M. and Crnic, L. S. (1996). Increased anxiety behaviors in autoimmune mice. *Behav. Neurosci.,* 110, 492 - 502.

[30] Liu, Y., Ho, R. C. and Mak, A. (2012). The role of interleukin (IL)-17 in anxiety and depression of patients with rheumatoid arthritis. *International Journal of Rheumatic Diseases,* 15 (2), 183 - 187.

[31] Figueiredo-Braga, M., Mota-Garcia, F., O'Connor, J. E., Garcia, J. R., Mota-Cardoso, R., Cardoso, C. S. and de Sousa, M. (2009). Cytokinesand anxiety in systemic lupus erythematosus (SLE) patients not receivingantidepressant medication: a little-explored frontier and some of its briefhistory. *Ann. N Y Acad. Sci.,* 1173, 286 - 291.

[32] Glaser, R., Sheridan, J., Malarkey, W. B., MacCallum, R. C., Kiecolt-Glaser, J. K. (2000). Chronic stress modulates the immune response to a pneumococcal pneumonia vaccine. *Psychosom. Med.,* 62, 804 - 807.

[33] Jabaaij, L., van Hattum, J., Vingerhoets, J. J., Oostveen, F. G., Duivenvoorden, H. J. and Ballieux, R. E. (1996). Modulation of immune response to rDNA hepatitis B vaccination by psychological stress. *J. Psychosom. Res.,* 41, 129 - 137.

[34] Morag, M., Morag, A., Reichenberg, A., Lerer, B. and Yirmiya, R. (1999). Psychological variables as predictors of rubella antibody titers and fatigue—a prospective, double blind study. *J. Psychiatr. Res.,* 33, 389 - 395.

[35] Burns, V. E., Drayson, M., Ring, C. and Carroll, D. (2002). Perceived stress and psychological well-being are associated with antibody status after meningitis C conjugate vaccination. *Psychosom. Med.,* 64, 963 - 970.

[36] Vedhara, K., Cox, N. K., Wilcock, G. K., Perks, P., Hunt, M., Anderson, S., Lightman, S. L. and Shanks, N. M. (1999). Chronic stress in elderly carers of dementia patients and antibody response to influenza vaccination. *Lancet,* 353, 627 - 631.

[37] Vedhara, K., McDermott, M. P., Evans, T. G., Treanor, J. J., Plummer, S., Tallon, D., Cruttenden, K. A. and Schifitto, G. (2002).

Chronic stress in nonelderly caregivers: psychological, endocrine and immune implications. *J. Psychosom. Res.,* 53, 1153 - 1161.
[38] Miller, G. E., Cohen, S., Pressman, S., Barkin, A., Rabin, B. S. and Treanor, J. J. (2004) Psychological stress and antibody response to influenza vaccination: when is the critical period for stress, and how does it get inside the body? *Psychosom. Med.,* 66, 215 - 223.
[39] Wittchen, H. U. (2002). Generalized anxiety disorder: prevalence, burden, and cost to society. *Depress. Anxiety,* 16, 162 - 171.
[40] Vieira, M. M., Ferreira, T. B., Pacheco, P. A., Barros, P. O., Almeida, C. R., Araújo-Lima, C. F., Silva-Filho, R. G., Hygino, J., Andrade, R. M., Linhares, U. C., Andrade, A. F. and Bento, C. A. (2010). Enhanced Th17 phenotype in individuals with generalized anxiety disorder. *J. Neuroimmunol.,* 229, 212 - 218.
[41] Barros, P. O., Ferreira, T. B., Vieira, M. M., Almeida, C. R., Araújo-Lima, C. F., Silva-Filho, R. G., Hygino, J., Andrade, R. M., Andrade, A. F. and Bento, C. A. (2011). Substance P enhances Th17 phenotype in individuals with generalized anxiety disorder: an event resistant to glucocorticoid inhibition. *J. Clin. Immunol.,* 31, 51 - 59.
[42] Bankier, B., Barajas, J., Martinez-Rumayor, A. and Januzzi, J. L. (2008). Association between C-reactive protein and generalized anxiety disorder in stable coronary heart disease patients. *Eur. Heart J.,* 29, 2212 - 2217.
[43] Ogłodek, E. A., Szota, A. M. and Just, M. J. (2015).The MCP-1, CCL-5 and SDF-1 chemokines as pro-inflammatory markers in generalized anxiety disorder and personality disorders. *Pharmacol. Rep.,* 67,85 - 9.
[44] Lenze, E. J., Mantella, R. C., Shi, P., Goate, A. M., Nowotny, P., Butters, M. A., Andreescu, C., Thompson, P. A. and Rollman, B. L. (2011). Elevated cortisol in older adults with generalized anxiety disorder is reduced by treatment: a placebo-controlled evaluation of escitalopram. *American Journal of Geriatric Psychiatry,* 19 (5), 482 - 490.
[45] Tafet, G. E., Feder, D. J., Abulafia, D. P., Roffman, S. S. (2005). Regulation of hypothalamic-pituitary-adrenal activity in response to

cognitive therapy in patients with generalized anxiety disorder. *Cognitive, Affective, and Behavioral Neuroscience,* 5 (1), 37 - 40.
[46] Steudte, S., Kirschbaum, C., Gao, W., Alexander, N., Schönfeld, S., Hoyer, J., Stalder, T. (2013). Hair cortisol as a biomarker of traumatization in healthy individuals and posttraumatic stress disorder patients. *Biological Psychiatry,* 74 (9), 639 - 646.
[47] Stein, M. B. and Stein, D. J. (2008). Social anxiety disorder. *The Lancet,* 371 (9618), 1115 - 1125.
[48] Russ, S. J., Herbert, J., Cooper, P., Gunnar, M. R., Goodyer, I., Croudace, T. and Murray, L. (2012). Cortisol levels in response to starting school in children at increased risk for social phobia. *Psychoneuroendocrinology,* 37 (4), 462 - 474.
[49] Garcia-Leal, C., Parente, A. C., Del-Ben, C. M., Guimarães, F. S., Moreira, A. C., Elias, L. L., Graeff, F. G. (2005). Anxiety and salivary cortisol in symptomatic and nonsymptomatic panic patients and healthy volunteers performing simulated public speaking. *Psychiatry Research,* 133 (2 - 3), 239 - 252.
[50] Bandelow, B., Wedekind, D., Sandvoss, V., Broocks, A., Hajak, G., Pauls, J., Peter, H. and Ruther, E. (2000). Diurnal variation of cortisol in panic disorder. *Psychiatry Research,* 95, 245 - 250.
[51] Brambilla, F., Bellodi, L., Perna, G., Bertani, A., Panerai, A. and Sacerdote, P. (1994). Plasma interleukin-1 beta concentrations in panic disorder. *Psychiatry Res.,* 54: 135 - 142.
[52] Koh, K. B. and Lee, Y. (2004). Reduced anxiety level by therapeutic interventions and cellmediated immunity in panic disorder patients. *Psychotherapy and Psychosomatics,* 73 (5), 286 - 292.
[53] Roelofs, K., van Peer, J., Berretty, E., de Jong, P., Spinhoven, P. and Elzinga, B. M. (2009). Hypothalamus-pituitary-adrenal axis hyperresponsiveness is associated with increased social avoidance behavior in social phobia. *Biological Psychiatry,* 65 (4), 336 - 343.
[54] Kawamura, N., Kim, Y. and Asukai, N. (2001). Suppression of cellular immunity in men with a past history of posttraumatic stress disorder. *American Journal of Psychiatry,* 158, 484 - 486.

[55] Baker, D. G., Nievergelt, C. M. and O'Connor, D. T. (2012). Biomarkers of PTSD: neuropeptides and immune signaling. *Neuropharmacology,* 62(2), 663 - 73.

[56] Rohleder, N., Joksimovic, L., Wolf, J. M. and Kirschbaum, C. (2004). Hypocortisolism and increased glucocorticoid sensitivity of pro-Inflammatory cytokine production in Bosnian war refugees with posttraumatic stress disorder. *Biol. Psychiatry,* 55, 745 - 751.

[57] Pace, T. W. and Heim, C. M. (2011). A short review on the psychoneuroimmunology of posttraumatic stress disorder: from risk factors to medical comorbidities. *Brain Behav. Immun.,* 25, 6 - 13.

[58] Wahbeh, H. and Oken, B. S. (2013). Salivary cortisol lower in posttraumatic stress disorder. *Journal of Traumatic Stress*, 26 (2), 241 - 248.

[59] Eraly, S. A., Nievergelt, C. M., Maihofer, A. X., Barkauskas, D. A., Biswas, N., Agorastos, A., O'Connor, D. T., Baker, D. G. and Marine Resiliency Study Team (2014). Assessment of plasma C-reactive protein as a biomarker of posttraumatic stress disorder risk. *JAMA Psychiatry*, 71 (4), 423 - 431.

[60] McCanlies, Erin C., Sewit Kesete Araia, Parveen Nedra Joseph, Anna Mnatsakanova, Michael E. Andrew, Cecil M. Burchfiel and John M. Violanti. (2011). "C-reactive protein, interleukin-6, and posttraumatic stress disorder symptomology in urban police officers". *Cytokine,* 55(1), 74 - 78.

[61] Gill, J., Vythilingam, M. and Page, G. G. (2008). Low cortisol, high DHEA, and high levels of stimulated TNF-alpha, and IL-6 in women with PTSD. *J. Trauma Stress*, 21(6), 530 - 9.

[62] Dekel, S., Ein-Dor, T., Gordon, K. M., Rosen, J. B. and Bonanno, G. A. (2013). Cortisol and PTSD symptoms among male and female high-exposure 9/11 survivors. *Journal of Traumatic Stress*, 26 (5), 6621 - 6625.

[63] Denys, D., Fluitman, S., Kavelaars, A., Heijnen, C. and Westenberg, H. (2004). Decreased TNF-alpha and NK activity in obsessive-compulsive disorder. *Psychoneuroendocrinology,* 29, 945 - 952.

[64] Fluitman, S., Denys, D., Vulink, N., Schutters, S., Heijnen, C. and Westenberg, H. (2010). Lipopolysaccharide-induced cytokine production in obsessive compulsive disorder and generalized social anxiety disorder. *Psychiatry Res.,* 178, 313 - 316.

[65] Monteleone, P., Catapano, F., Fabrazzo, M., Tortorella, A. and Maj, M. (1998). Decreased blood levels of tumor necrosis factor-alpha in patients with obsessive-compulsive disorder. *Neuropsychobiology,* 37, 182 - 185.

[66] Carpenter, L. L., Heninger, G. R., McDougle, C. J., Tyrka, A. R., Epperson, C. N. and Price, L. H. (2002). Cerebrospinal fluid interleukin-6 in obsessive-compulsive disorder and trichotillomania. *Psychiatry Res.,* 112, 257 - 262.

[67] Konuk, N., Tekin, I. O., Ozturk, U., Atik, L., Atasoy, **N.**, Bektas, S. and Erdogan, A. (2007). Plasma levels of tumor necrosis factor-alpha and interleukin-6 in obsessive compulsive disorder. *Mediators Inflamm.,* 2007, 65704.

In: Depression and Anxiety
Editor: Shelley L. Becker

ISBN: 978-1-53617-229-4
© 2020 Nova Science Publishers, Inc.

Chapter 5

PSYCHOPHYSIOLOGICAL MEASURES OF ANXIETY

Suprakash Chaudhury[1,*], Swaleha Mujawar[1] and Daniel Saldanha[1]

Department of Psychiatry, Dr. D. Y. Patil Medical College,
Dr. D. Y. Patil University, Pune,
Maharshtra, India

ABSTRACT

This chapter uses pooled data from 1983-2008 to assess the psychophysiological measures of anxiety. Various databases were searched for articles in English using search words of psychophysiological measures of anxiety, markers for anxiety, physiological changes anxiety, and monitors of emotional change. A total of 76 articles were screened and the bibliographies of all relevant articles were searched for further publications. It was found that anxiety leads to sympathetic over-activity which can be measured by heart-rate, blood-pressure electroencephalogram etc. Loudness of the auditory evoked potential measures activity in the primary auditory cortex in response to

---

[*] Corresponding Author's Email: suprakashch@gmail.com.

different tone intensities and is inversely proportional to serotonergic activity. Patients with anxiety disorders have reduced heart rate variability. The serotonin transporter promoter polymorphism is another measure. Individuals carrying one or two copies of the 's' form had reduction in 5-HTT availability and were associated with increased anxiety. The implications of the findings will contribute to further research and development of better management for anxiety disorders.

Keywords: psychophysiological measures of anxiety, physiological changes anxiety, monitors of emotional change

INTRODUCTION

Psychophysiology is the study of relationships between psychological events and brain responses. It is concerned with the physiological bases of psychological processes. It is derived from the Greek word psȳkhē meaning "breath, life, soul" and physis meaning "nature, origin". Even though psychophysiology as a field was not part of the mainstream psychological and medical science during the 1960 and 1970s, in recent times, this science has found itself placed at the crossroads of psychology and medicine, and its recognition and significance has increased with the realization of mind-body inter-relatedness.

PSYCHOPHYSIOLOGICAL PARAMETERS

Psychophysiological parameters can be measured as behaviour, reports and readings [1].

Behaviour is measured by observing and recording actual actions, such as running, eye movements, and facial expressions. However, they are not frequently used in human studies though these are easy to record in animals. The report measures include self-ratings of psychological states and introspection by the subject [2], or measuring the bodily awareness such as heartbeat detection [3]. The self-report measures have a number of advantages like an importance on correctly understanding individual experience and their perception. However, there are also disadvantages like the chances of not correctly understanding a scale or not recalling events correctly [4]. The readings involve measuring visceral events with the help of instrument. The following can be recorded: cardiovascular measures like cardiac output, heart rate (HR), beats per minute (BPM); heart rate variability (HRV); cardiodynamics, recorded via impedance cardiography, EEG (electroencephalography) or brain waves, electrogastrogram (EGG), fMRI (functional magnetic resonance imaging), electro dermal activity which is a standardized term encompassing skin conductance response (SCR), and galvanic skin response (GSR), vasomotor activity, muscle tension, electromyography (EMG) which measures the muscle activity, alteration in pupil diameter with thought and emotion (pupillometry), and eye movements recorded via the electro-oculogram (EOG) and direction-of-gaze methods. The advantage of these measures is that they provide a precise and objective data which is perceiver-independent. However, it should be kept in mind that basal levels of arousal and responsiveness may be different among different people and may differ with different situations and also that any motion or physical activity can affect and change the responses [5].

USES OF PSYCHOPHYSIOLOGICAL MEASURES

These measures are used to evaluate attention and emotional responses to certain stimuli, during physical exertion, and also to understand clearly the thinking practices. Physiological sensors have been employed to measure emotions in schools [6] as well as intelligent educational organizations [7]. It has been proven that emotional incidents are in part made up of physiological reactions [8]. Studies which have found a correlation between emotions and psychophysiology started with finding consistent autonomic nervous system (ANS) responses and then associating them to the precise emotion. Anger is associated with a few physiological changes such as high cardiac output and raised diastolic blood pressure. This can help recognize different forms of emotions and also predict the emotional responses. Consistent patterns of ANS responses that were associated with specific emotions under different situations have been established. Paul Ekman et al. reported that the emotion-specific changes in the ANS were produced by reliving previous emotional encounters and by creating facial prototypes of emotion muscle by muscle. This autonomic change produced differentiated between positive and negative emotions and also between different negative emotions [9]. It was observed that there was a greater variability in the ANS changes to distinct emotion inductions in individuals and also as time progressed in the same individuals, and more so between social groups [10]. These variations can be explained by the variations in classification of stimuli, context of the research, or induction technique, causing variability in documented emotional response or situation. Nevertheless, it was also observed that characteristics of the subject could also alter ANS changes. Factors which can alter physiological responses in a laboratory setting include learned or conditioned responses to various provocations, the level of arousal at the start of experiment or in between test recovery, and characteristic attentiveness of the subject [11]. It should be noted that fear may have subtypes such as freezing or fleeing, both of which have been observed to have discrete physiological patterns and theoretically different neuronal circuits [12].

PSYCHOPHYSIOLOGICAL MARKERS USED TO STUDY ANXIETY DISORDERS

The psychophysiological markers that have been used to study dysfunctional neural, serotonergic, cognitive and autonomic activities associated with anxiety disorders include:

- Measures of autonomic nervous system
- Loudness dependence of the auditory evoked potential

- Event-Related Potentials
- Heart Rate Variability (HRV)
- Genetic polymorphisms
- Amygdala hyperactivity and dysfunctional prefrontal activity

Measures of Autonomic Nervous System

- Since anxiety leads to sympathetic over-activity, it can be measured by increase in the following: blood-pressure, pulse rate, respiration rate, salivation, pupil size, skin conductance or palmar sweating, electromyogram, electroencephalogram.
- These measures revert to normal values as soon as anxiety is alleviated [13].

Loudness of the Auditory Evoked Potential

- It measures activity in the primary auditory cortex in response to different tone intensities and is a marker for the functioning of the central serotonergic system
- It is inversely proportional to central serotonergic activity
- It has been utilized to study dysfunctional serotonergic and dopaminergic activity in patients with generalised anxiety disorder[14, 15].

Event-Related Potentials

P1:
- These are the initial main voltage deflection which are positive and occur 50 to 165 milliseconds after the exposure to stimulus and the early posterior negativities (EPNs) which show negative deflection

over the temporo-occipital areas in the time window between 150 to 300 milliseconds after exposure to emotional stimuli
- The people at risk for anxiety show an increased early P1 component to fearful faces compared to neutral faces at occipital electrode areas
- Nonetheless, they do not show more EPNs in reaction to fearful faces indicating attentional evasion subsequent to the preliminary attentional vigilance or the inability to discriminate the non-threat stimuli from threating ones. [16, 17]

P2:
- The major positive voltage deflection occurring 50-165 milliseconds after the onset of stimulus
- High-trait anxiety participants have greater amplitudes of the P2 component to angry faces
- Higher P2 components signify higher attentional allotment to threat-related stimuli, which is commonly seen in people suffering from anxiety disorders.

Error-Related Negativity

- These can be seen as a negative deflection at fronto-central areas and areproduced in the anterior cingulate cortex at the time when an erroneous response is made. It is found to peak at 50 to100 milliseconds after exposure to stimulus
- Larger Error-related negativity (ERN) component has been associated with anxiety
- Administrating anxiolytics such as oxazepam and alprazolam has decreased ERN amplitudes
- Error monitoring function of the anterior cingulate cortex seen by the ERN may play a part as an endophenotype of anxiety disorders[18, 19].

Heart Rate Variability

- It is the difference in beat-to-beat changes in the heart rate. It gives a hint of the interaction between parasympathetic (vagal) and sympathetic activity.
- Under resting conditions, the heart is predominantly under the control of parasympathetic activity.
- A low HRV shows dysregulation in the autonomic system. It is associated with raised sympathetic activity and decreased vagal activity of the heart.
- Patients with anxiety disorders have reduced heart rate variability
- It is seen in panic disorder, generalized anxiety disorder, and even children of patients with panic disorder [20, 21].

Genetic Predispositions in Anxiety Disorders

Genetic predispositions seen in anxiety disorders are as follows:

The serotonin transport promoter polymorphism:
- The serotonin producing raphe neurons project to various brain areas like the amygdala, cerebral cortex and hippocampus. They integrate functions namely cognition, motor function, emotion, pain, circadian and neuroendocrine functions such as appetite, sleep and sex.
- The serotonin transporter (5-HTT) has a major function in controlling serotonin neurotransmission by aiding the reuptake of serotonin from the synaptic cleft
- Two different alleles are produced due to polymorphism in the promoter region of the serotonin transporter gene. They are called 's' for the short allele and 'l' for the long allele.
- People having one or two copies of the 's' form were seen to have a decrease in serotonin and were witnessed to have more anxiety-

related behaviors and more chances of developing anxiety in demanding life circumstances [22, 23].

Catechol-O-methyltransferase (COMT):
o COMT is an enzyme that metabolizes brain dopamine and norepinephrine
o Its gene is present on chromosome 22q11. This site has many single nucleotide polymorphisms that are important from functional point of view. One of these Val158Met modulates the COMT activity in the prefrontal cortex. It is seen to encode either valine (Val) or methionine (Met) .Val158Met may be linked with anxiety disorders[24, 25].

Brain-derived neurotrophic factor (BDNF):
o BDNF functions in synaptic plasticity, neuronal growth and differentiation.
o It is also observed to mediate the effects of stress
o Decreased BDNF expression in the hippocampus was seen in response to stress, which may cause hippocampus-dependent memory problems and reduced hippocampal volume found in subjects suffering from post-traumatic stress disorder [26, 27].

Amygdala Hyperactivity and Reduced PFC Function

- Anxiety disorders are linked with hyperactivity of the amygdala
- People with anxiety have reduced activity in anterior cingulate cortex (ACC) and lateral prefrontal cortex
- It was seen that successful treatment in subjects with social phobia lead to decreased amygdala activity as shown by functional magnetic resonance imaging (fMRI) studies [28-30].

The clinical uses of the measures are as follows:

1. *Biofeedback*: It is the practice of achieving better awareness of various physiological functions mainly by using different instruments that supply evidence on the activity of those same systems, with the objective of the patient being able to control them at will. It has shown promising results in treating anxiety disorders.
2. *Research*: These measures are useful in research for the development of newer drugs and also finding out the etiological factors in anxiety.

CONCLUSION

The psychophysiological markers are useful to study dysfunctional neural, serotonergic, cognitive and autonomic activities associated with anxiety disorders. They can be measures of autonomic nervous system, loudness dependence of the auditory evoked potential, event-related potentials, heart rate variability (HRV), genetic polymorphisms, amygdala hyperactivity and dysfunctional prefrontal activity. They have a variety of clinical uses in biofeedback and research. The physiological measures of anxiety can guide us towards better diagnosis and treatment and should be used clinically in common practice.Even though there is a lot of research being done in this field, there is a greater scope for further research in this area and should be encouraged by clinicians.

REFERENCES

[1] Cacioppo, John, Tassinary, Louis, Berntson, Gary (2007). "25". *Handbook of Psychophysiology* (3rd ed.). Cambridge: Cambridge University Press. pp. 581 - 607.

[2] Bradley, M. and Lang, P. (1994). Measuring Emotion: The Self-Assessment Manikin and the Semantic Differential. *Journal of Behavior Therapy and Experimental Psychiatry*, 25 (1): 49 - 59.

[3] Weins, S., Mezzacappa, E. and Katkin, E. (2000). Heartbeat Detection and the Experience of Emotions. *Cognition and Emotion*, 14 (3): 417 - 427.

[4] Robinson, M. and Clore, G. (2002). Episodic and Semantic Knowledge in Emotional Self-Report: Evidence for Two Judgment Processes. *Journal of Personality and Social Psychology*, 83 (1): 198 - 215.

[5] Glynn, L., Christenfeld, N. and Gerin, W. (2002). The Role of Rumination in Recovery From Reactivity; Cardiovascular Consequences of Emotional States. *Psychosomatic Medicine*, 64 (5): 714 - 726.

[6] Arroyo, I., Woolf, B., Cooper, D., Burleson, W., Muldner, K. and Christopherson, R. (2009). Emotion Sensors Go to School. *Artificial Intelligence in Education*, 1 (1): 18 - 37.

[7] Hussain, M. Sazzad, Omar AlZoubi, Rafael A. Calvo and Sidney K. D'Mello. (2011). Affect detection from multichannel physiology during learning sessions with AutoTutor. *In International Conference on Artificial Intelligence in Education*. Berlin, Heidelberg: Springer. pp. 131 - 138.

[8] Williams, J. (1884). What is an Emotion? *Mind*, 34 (2): 188 - 205.

[9] Paul, E., Levenson, R. and Friesen, W. (1983). Autonomic Nervous System Activity Distinguishes among Emotions. *Science*, 221 (4616): 1208 - 1210.

[10] Cacioppo, J., Berntson, G., Larsen, J., Poehlmann, K. and Ito, T. (2000). The Psychophysiology of Emotion. *Handbook of Emotions*, 2: 173 - 191.

[11] Stemmler, G. and Wacker, J. (2010). Personality, Emotion, and Individual Differences in Physiological Responses. *Biological Psychology*, 84 (3): 541 - 551.

[12] Gross, C. and Canteras, N. (2012). The Many Paths to Fear. *Nature Reviews Neuroscience*, 13 (9): 651 - 658.

[13] Lader, M. (1983). The neuropsychology of anxiety. *Personality and Individual Differences*, 4(6):720.
[14] Hegerl, U. and Juckel, G. (1993). Intensity dependence of auditory evoked potentials as an indicator of central serotonergic neurotransmission: a new hypothesis. *Biological psychiatry*, 1; 33(3):173 - 87.
[15] Juckel, G., Hegerl, U., Molár, M., Csépe, V. and Karmos, G. (1999). Auditory evoked potentials reflect serotonergic neuronal activity-a study in behaving cats administered drugs acting on 5-HT1A autoreceptors in the dorsal raphe nuclesus. *Neuropsychopharmacology*, 21(6):710 - 6.
[16] Schupp, Harald T., Tobias Flaisch, Jessica Stockburger and Markus Junghöfer (2006). Emotion and attention: event-related brain potential studies. *Progress in Brain Research*, 156: 31 - 51.
[17] Holmes, A., Nielsen, M. K. and Green, S. (2008). Effects of anxiety on the processing of fearful and happy faces: An event-related potential study. *Biological Psychology*, 77(2):159 - 173.
[18] Olvet, Doreen M. and Greg Hajcak (2008). The error-related negativity (ERN) and psychopathology: Toward an endophenotype. *Clinical Psychology Review*, 28(8): 1343 - 1354.
[19] Xiao Zeping, Jijun Wang, Ming Zhang, Hui Li, Yingying Tang, Yuan Wang, Qing Fan and John A. Fromson (2011). Error-related negativity abnormalities in generalized anxiety disorder and obsessive–compulsive disorder. *Progress in Neuro-Psychopharmacology and Biological Psychiatry*, 35(1) 265 - 272.
[20] Friedman, Bruce H. (2007). An autonomic flexibility–neurovisceral integration model of anxiety and cardiac vagal tone. *Biological Psychology*, 74(2), 185 - 199.
[21] Srinivasan, K., Ashok, M. V., Vaz, M. and Yeragani, V. K. (2002). Decreased chaos of heart rate time series in children of patients with panic disorder. *Depression and Anxiety*, 15, 159 - 167.
[22] Lesch, Klaus-Peter, Dietmar Bengel, Armin Heils, Sue Z. Sabol, Benjamin D. Greenberg, Susanne Petri, Jonathan Benjamin, Clemens R. Müller, Dean H. Hamer and Dennis L. Murphy (1996).

Association of anxiety-related traits with a polymorphism in the serotonin transporter gene regulatory region. *Science,* 274, no. 5292, 1527 - 1531.

[23] Hariri, A. R., Venkata, S. M., Tessitore, A., Bhaskar, K., Fera, F., Goldman, D., Egan, M. F. and Weinberger, D. R. (2002). Serotonin transporter genetic variation and the response of the human amygdala. *Science,* 297, no. 5580, 400 - 403.

[24] Funke, B., Malhotra, A. K., Finn, C. T., Plocik, A. M., Lake, S. L., Lencz, T., DeRosse, P., Kane, J. M. and Kucherlapati, R. (2005). *Behavioral and Brain Functions,* 1(19), 1 - 9.

[25] Harrison, Paul J. and Elizabeth M. Tunbridge (2008). "Catechol-O-methyltransferase (COMT): a gene contributing to sex differences in brain function, and to sexual dimorphism in the predisposition to psychiatric disorders". *Neuropsychopharmacology,* 33(13), 3037.

[26] Chen, Z. Y., Jing, D., Bath, K. G., Ieraci, A., Khan, T., Siao, C. J., Herrera, D. G. et al. (2006). Genetic variant BDNF (Val66Met) polymorphism alters anxiety-related behavior. *Science,* 314, no. 5796, 140 - 143.

[27] Gadow, K. D., Roohi, J., DeVincent, C. J., Kirsch, S. and Hatchwell, E. (2009). Association of COMT (Val158Met) and BDNF (Val66Met) gene polymorphisms with anxiety, ADHD and tics in children with autism spectrum disorder. *Journal of Autism and Developmental Disorders,* 39, 1542 - 1551.

[28] Yair, B. H., Lamy, D. and Glickman. S. (2005). Attentional bias in anxiety: A behavioral and ERP study. *Brain and Cognition,* 59, 11 - 22.

[29] Bishop, S., Duncan, J., Brett, M. and Lawrence, A. D. (2004). Prefrontal cortical function and anxiety: controlling attention to threat-related stimuli. *Nature Neuroscience,* 7, 184 - 188.

[30] Kilts, C. D., Kelsey, J. E., Knight, B., Ely, T. D., Bowman, F. D., Gross, R. E., Selvig, A., Gordon, A., Newport, D. J. and Nemeroff, C. B. (2006). The neural correlates of social anxiety disorder and response to pharmacotherapy. *Neuropsychopharmacology,* 31, 2243 - 2253.

INDEX

A

active inference, 14, 15, 16, 17, 19, 20, 21, 24, 25, 28, 30, 34, 37, 42
acute stress, 25, 49, 105, 113
adaptation, 8, 10, 18, 20, 25, 28, 31, 37, 50, 53, 96
ADHD, 18, 134
adolescents, 5, 9, 108
adrenocorticotropic hormone, 65, 106
adults, 44, 78, 87, 99, 100, 101, 108, 113, 118
adverse effects, ix, 58, 66, 74, 78
aetiology, 63, 68
affective disorder, 77
age, ix, x, 45, 47, 58, 63, 80, 84, 87, 88, 89, 90, 91, 92, 95, 109, 120
alcohol withdrawal, 86
allostasis, 2, 7, 8, 9, 18, 20, 22, 25, 27, 30, 31, 35, 42, 49
amygdala, 106, 129, 130, 131, 134
anorgasmia, 62, 63, 65
anterior cingulate cortex, 34, 107, 128, 130

antidepressant(s), viii, ix, 2, 43, 44, 57, 58, 65, 66, 67, 72, 73, 74, 75, 76, 77, 78, 80, 81, 84, 86, 87, 95, 97, 98, 99, 102
antidepressant medication, 44, 80
antihypertensive agents, 64
antipsychotic drugs, 97
anxiety, vii, ix, x, xi, xii, 4, 10, 28, 30, 31, 32, 43, 45, 47, 50, 51, 64, 70, 84, 85, 86, 87, 88, 89, 90, 91, 92, 93, 94, 95, 97, 98, 99, 101, 103, 104, 105, 106, 107, 108, 109, 110, 111, 113, 114, 115, 117, 118, 119, 121, 123, 124, 126, 127, 128, 129, 130, 131, 133, 134
anxiety disorder(s), vii, viii, ix, x, xi, xii, 32, 43, 47, 70, 84, 85, 86, 87, 88, 89, 90, 91, 92, 93, 94, 97, 99, 104, 107, 108, 111, 114, 118, 119, 121, 124, 126, 127, 128, 129, 130, 131, 133, 134
arousal, 28, 61, 62, 63, 64, 67, 68, 70, 71, 73, 79, 125, 126
asymptomatic, 105, 110, 114
auditory cortex, xii, 123, 127
auditory evoked potentials, 133
autism, 18, 49, 134

autonomic nervous system, 68, 125, 126, 131
avoidance, 20, 25, 61, 111, 119
avoidance behavior, 119

B

Bayesian, 14, 15, 20, 32, 37, 38, 41, 44, 46, 49, 50, 55
behavior therapy, 50
behavioral change, 42, 48
behaviors, 20, 24, 33, 97, 117, 130
benzodiazepine, vii, 86, 98, 100
brain, 11, 13, 15, 16, 17, 18, 19, 20, 21, 23, 24, 25, 27, 28, 29, 32, 36, 43, 44, 45, 48, 50, 51, 52, 105, 106, 107, 115, 124, 125, 129, 130, 133, 134
brain activity, 16
brain functioning, 13

C

central nervous system (CNS), 106, 113, 114
cerebral cortex, 106, 129
children, 9, 108, 110, 114, 119, 129, 133, 134
clinical depression, 6, 10, 20
cognitive therapy, 5, 33, 44, 46, 109, 113, 119
cognitive-behavioral therapy, 97
conditioned response, 63, 126
conversion disorder, 37
coping strategies, 97
coronary artery disease, 76
coronary heart disease, 108, 118
cortical neurons, 16
corticotropin, 65, 106
cortisol, vii, xi, 8, 103, 104, 106, 107, 108, 109, 110, 111, 112, 113, 118, 119, 120
cultural influence, 65, 66

cytokine(s), 106, 107, 108, 111, 113, 115, 116, 120, 121

D

deep brain stimulation, 34
dependence, vii, ix, x, xi, 84, 85, 86, 87, 88, 89, 90, 92, 93, 94, 95, 97, 98, 100, 101, 126, 131, 133
depression, vii, viii, ix, x, xi, 1, 2, 3, 4, 5, 6, 8, 9, 10, 11, 12, 18, 19, 20, 21, 22, 24, 25, 27, 28, 29, 31, 32, 33, 34, 36, 37, 40, 41, 42, 43, 44, 45, 46, 47, 48, 49, 50, 51, 53, 54, 57, 58, 59, 64, 66, 68, 70, 71, 73, 74, 76, 78, 84, 85, 86, 87, 88, 89, 90, 91, 92, 93, 94, 95, 98, 100, 101, 104, 111, 113, 114, 115, 116, 117
depressive symptoms, 10, 28, 36, 49, 68, 72, 77
despair, 6, 9
Diagnostic and Statistical Manual of Mental Disorders, 60, 104, 114
distress, 60, 61, 62, 63, 65
dopamine, 9, 34, 50, 67, 68, 74, 107, 115, 130
dopamine agonist, 74
dopaminergic, 18, 127
drugs, 64, 67, 73, 77, 86, 87, 97, 131, 133
DSM, 104, 111
DSM-IV-TR, 65
dynamic systems, 29
dynamical systems, 16
dyspareunia, 72
dysthymia, 11

E

emotion, 4, 9, 32, 96, 125, 129
emotional responses, 96, 125
emotional stimuli, 128
emotionality, 116

environmental factors, 63
environmental impact, 19
environmental stress, 7, 53
event-related potential, 131, 133
evoked potential, xii, 123, 126, 131, 133
evolution, 2, 41
external environment, 19
eye movement, 39, 124

F

facial expression, 124
fear, 110, 126
feelings, 9, 35
female sexual dysfunction, viii, 57, 58, 59, 61, 63, 69, 70, 71, 73, 80, 81
fMRI, 125, 130
free energy, 2, 16, 18, 21, 22, 25, 32, 45
Freud, 5, 45

G

generalized anxiety disorder, ix, x, 84, 87, 88, 89, 104, 108, 118, 119, 129, 133
generative model, 13, 15, 16, 17, 19, 20, 21, 22, 29, 34, 35, 37, 38, 41
genetic polymorphisms, 131
glucocorticoid(s), 106, 115, 118, 120
glutamate, 107, 116
goal attainment, 30

H

hallucinations, 46, 51
heart rate (HR), xii, 22, 25, 124, 125, 129, 131, 133
helplessness, 3, 24, 52
hippocampus, 106, 129, 130
hopelessness, 3, 6, 35

HPA axis, 11, 104, 105, 106, 107, 110, 111, 112, 113
hyperactivity, 127, 130, 131
hyperarousal, 28
hypercholesterolemia, 73
hypersomnia, 4, 10, 28
hypertension, 8, 19
hyperthyroidism, 8
hypothalamus, 106
hypothyroidism, 8
hysteria, 44

I

IFN, 106, 108
IL-17, 107
IL-8, 111
immune activation, 104
immune function, 104, 105, 111, 114
immune memory, 11
immune response, 105, 117
immune system, 30, 104, 106, 108, 113, 115
immunosuppression, 104, 111
information processing, 13, 39, 40
information processing theory, 40
inhibition, 8, 9, 15, 52, 60, 79, 118
inhibitor, 65, 67, 73, 80, 81
insomnia, xi, 10, 28, 85, 86, 87, 92, 95, 97, 99, 101
interferon, 105, 106, 111
interferon-γ, 106
internal consistency, 89
internal environment, 7, 13, 26
intervention, 33, 34, 37, 38, 39, 97
introspection, 124

L

learned helplessness, 5, 24
libido, 30, 63, 64, 67, 70, 72, 73
lichen planus, 72

loss of appetite, 8, 10, 20, 30
loss of libido, 65
lymphocytes, 111, 112

M

magnetic resonance imaging, 125, 130
major depression, vii, ix, x, xi, 2, 11, 24, 36, 43, 44, 47, 53, 76, 84, 85, 87, 88, 89, 90, 91, 93, 94, 95, 101, 115, 116
major depressive disorder, 47, 50, 52, 79, 97, 100
MCP-1, 108, 118
medication, 60, 65, 71, 72, 73, 78, 101, 117
medicine, 41, 45, 124
melatonin, 69, 79
memory, 11, 39, 74, 86, 116, 130
mental disorder, 3, 12, 41, 66
mental health, 12, 37, 88
mental illness, 65
mental representation, 22, 36
meta-analysis, 43, 73, 81, 98, 101
metabolism, 8, 25, 37, 50, 107
metabolized, 27
methylphenidate, 74
monitors of emotional change, viii, xii, 123, 124
monocyte chemoattractant protein, 108
mood disorder, 41
motivation, 8, 9, 18, 30, 33
motor stimulation, 39
mRNA, 7

N

necrosis, 105
negative emotions, 126
negativity, 128, 133
neurogenesis, 107, 116
neurological disease, 64
neuronal circuits, 126
neurons, 16, 18, 129
neuropeptides, 9, 105, 120
neurophysiology, 70
neuropsychology, 133
neurotransmission, 74, 129, 133
neurotransmitters, 68, 105
nitric oxide, 68, 79, 116
nitric oxide synthase, 79
non-pharmacological treatments, 97
norepinephrine, 130

O

obsessive-compulsive disorder (OCD), 104, 106, 112, 113, 120, 121
outpatient(s), x, 74, 75, 81, 84, 88, 100

P

panic attack, 110
panic disorder, ix, x, 84, 86, 87, 88, 89, 90, 100, 104, 119, 129, 133
parasympathetic activity, 129
pathology, 6, 8, 12, 37, 40
pathophysiology, 76, 79, 116
Pavlovian conditioning, 51
peripheral nervous system, 69
personality, 11, 18, 97, 105, 109, 118
personality disorder, 97, 109, 118
personality factors, 105
pharmacological agents, 72
pharmacological treatment, 98, 109
pharmacotherapy, 66, 134
phenotype(s), 8, 20, 31, 41, 108, 115, 118
physiological changes anxiety, viii, xii, 123, 124
pleasure, 8, 30, 33, 58, 60
postpartum depression, 5
posttraumatic stress, xi, 103, 105, 113, 119, 120

post-traumatic stress disorder (PTSD), 8, 18, 49, 55, 98, 104, 106, 111, 112, 113, 120, 130
precision weighting, 17, 18, 21, 22, 23, 24, 25, 32, 37, 38, 39
prediction error, 13, 14, 17, 20, 21, 23, 24, 27, 29, 30, 32, 34, 35, 37, 38, 39, 41
predictive coding, viii, 2, 4, 13, 18, 20, 34, 46
predictive processing, viii, 2, 13, 17, 41
priors, 15, 19, 20, 21, 22, 23, 24, 25, 26, 27, 28, 29, 30, 34, 35, 38, 39, 51
psychiatric disorders, 18, 108, 111, 134
psychiatric illness, 64, 106, 113
psychiatric patients, 88, 100
psychoanalysis, 5, 40, 45
psychobiology, 99
psychological problems, 62
psychological processes, 124
psychological states, 124
psychological stress, 8, 117
psychological well-being, 117
psychopathology, viii, 2, 6, 13, 18, 19, 34, 36, 40, 47, 67, 133
psychophysiological measures of anxiety, vii, xii, 123, 124
psychosis, 18, 42
psychosocial stress, 19
psychotherapy, 2, 3, 4, 35, 37, 38, 40, 41, 44, 48, 50, 52, 54, 55, 66, 96, 109
psychotropic medications, ix, 84, 86

Q

quality of life, vii, ix, 46, 58, 65, 66

R

reactions, 4, 18, 22, 38, 46, 105, 125
reactivity, 9, 11, 39

recovery, 6, 9, 11, 24, 25, 27, 28, 29, 30, 31, 32, 33, 45, 47, 65, 126
regression, x, xi, 85, 90, 93, 114
regression model, x, xi, 85, 93
relaxation, 62, 73, 97
remission, 48, 73, 86
response, viii, xii, 2, 4, 5, 6, 7, 8, 11, 12, 13, 14, 18, 19, 21, 25, 38, 40, 53, 70, 71, 80, 81, 96, 106, 117, 118, 119, 123, 125, 126, 127, 128, 130, 134
response time, 11

S

sadness, 9, 30
schizophrenia, 3, 42, 43, 113
sedative, ix, 84, 86, 95
self-control, 58
self-efficacy, 22, 23, 24, 25, 26, 27, 29, 31, 33, 35, 39
self-esteem, 64, 70
self-image, 71
self-inefficacy, 22, 24, 25, 27, 28, 30, 32, 35
sensation(s), 13, 26, 30, 32, 62, 68, 71
sensitivity, 31, 34, 35, 42, 47, 72, 120
serotonin, xii, 2, 34, 67, 68, 70, 73, 79, 80, 81, 107, 115, 124, 129, 134
sertraline, 77, 78
severe stress, 11
sex differences, 134
sexual abuse, 62
sexual activity, 61, 64, 79
sexual behaviour, 66, 69, 79
sexual contact, 61
sexual desire, 61, 62, 63, 64, 68, 72
sexual dimorphism, 134
sexual dysfunctions, ix, 58, 63, 67, 71
sexual experiences, 59, 64
sexual health, 59, 75
sexual intercourse, 58, 63

sexual problems, viii, 57, 63, 64, 65, 67, 68, 74
side effects, 66, 67, 73, 78
smoking cessation, 71
smooth muscle, 62, 69, 73
social anxiety, 45, 104, 121, 134
social environment, 20
social interaction, 48
social phobia, 119, 130
social resources, 5
social skills, 109
social withdrawal, 6, 8, 20
socioeconomic status, 87, 90
stimulation, 10, 27, 34, 39, 60, 62, 63, 65, 67, 107
stress, viii, xi, 2, 4, 6, 7, 8, 11, 12, 14, 19, 20, 21, 22, 23, 24, 25, 26, 30, 32, 35, 39, 40, 42, 48, 49, 50, 51, 52, 53, 71, 98, 103, 104, 105, 106, 107, 111, 113, 114, 117, 118, 119, 120, 130
stress response, 4, 6, 7, 8, 11, 12, 19, 20, 21, 22, 23, 25, 32, 40
stressors, 7, 25, 50
subjective experience, x, 85, 89
substance abuse, 89
suicidal behavior, 10, 53
suppression, 18, 21, 111
surgical intervention, 62
symptoms, viii, ix, xi, 1, 3, 4, 5, 8, 10, 28, 31, 32, 38, 42, 43, 47, 64, 72, 84, 85, 86, 87, 92, 93, 95, 96, 97, 106, 112, 115, 120

T

T cell, 108, 111, 113
T lymphocytes, 114
techniques, 38, 40, 71, 97, 106
testosterone, 68, 72
T-helper cell, 106, 111
therapeutic encounter, 37, 38, 39, 41
therapeutic interventions, 37, 119
therapy, viii, 2, 4, 10, 33, 34, 35, 36, 37, 38, 40, 41, 46, 48, 72, 76, 79
thoughts, 39, 61, 97, 108
TNF-alpha (TNF-α), 106, 107, 112, 113, 120
trauma, 9, 12, 32, 62, 69
treatment, vii, viii, ix, xi, xii, 1, 2, 3, 12, 32, 41, 44, 46, 58, 65, 67, 71, 72, 73, 74, 76, 81, 84, 85, 86, 88, 95, 96, 97, 99, 100, 101, 102, 104, 109, 111, 113, 115, 116, 118, 130, 131
trichotillomania, 121

U

underlying mechanisms, xi, 103

V

violence, 59, 112
vulnerability, 6, 99, 105

W

well-being, 59, 71
withdrawal, 6, 8, 9, 10, 11, 24, 25, 27, 29, 30, 31, 32, 33, 64, 65, 72, 79, 86
withdrawal symptoms, 86

Related Nova Publications

THE NEW SCIENCE OF CURIOSITY

AUTHOR: Goren Gordon

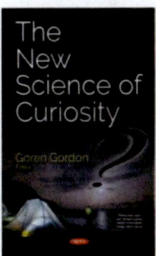

SERIES: Psychology of Emotions, Motivations and Actions

BOOK DESCRIPTION: Curiosity is the foundation of childhood development and continues on into adulthood; it is the cornerstone of scientific discovery, art and play. In the past, the study of curiosity has been mainly restricted to the field of psychology.

HARDCOVER ISBN: 978-1-53613-800-9
RETAIL PRICE: $195

UNDERSTANDING IMPULSIVE BEHAVIOR: ASSESSMENT, INFLUENCES AND GENDER DIFFERENCES

EDITOR: Christian Braddon

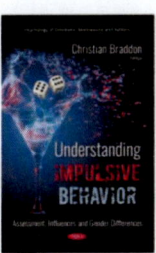

SERIES: Psychology of Emotions, Motivations and Actions

BOOK DESCRIPTION: In this compilation, the authors begin by describing the main impulsive behavior assessment instruments in animals and humans.

SOFTCOVER ISBN: 978-1-53613-815-3
RETAIL PRICE: $95

To see a complete list of Nova publications, please visit our website at www.novapublishers.com

Related Nova Publications

EMPATHY: PAST, PRESENT AND FUTURE PERSPECTIVES

EDITOR: Albert K. Bach

SERIES: Psychology of Emotions, Motivations and Actions

BOOK DESCRIPTION: In this compilation, the authors analyze the feeling of empathy in the context of the constitution of empathetic bonds that mark human relations. Empathy is shown as a spontaneous manifestation, natural and implicit, and present in all human encounters.

HARDCOVER ISBN: 978-1-53616-372-8
RETAIL PRICE: $230

THE PSYCHOLOGY OF RIVALRY

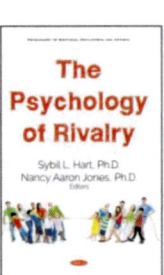

EDITORS: Sybil L. Hart, Ph.D. and Nancy Aaron Jones, Ph.D.

SERIES: Psychology of Emotions, Motivations and Actions

BOOK DESCRIPTION: *The Psychology of Rivalry* is an edited volume made up of chapters by leading researchers and theorists in the fields of psychology, human development, family studies, evolutionary psychology, behavioral neuroscience and genetics.

HARDCOVER ISBN: 978-1-53614-172-6
RETAIL PRICE: $230

To see a complete list of Nova publications, please visit our website at www.novapublishers.com